THE
BOWFLEX®
BODY PLAN

THE
BOWFLEX®
BODY PLAN

THE POWER IS YOURS
BUILD MORE MUSCLE • LOSE MORE FAT

ELLINGTON DARDEN, PH.D.

RODALE®

Notice

The information given here is designed to help you make informed decisions about your body and health. The suggestions for specific foods, nutritional supplements, and exercises in this program are not intended to replace appropriate or necessary medical care. If you have specific medical symptoms, consult your physician immediately. If any recommendations given in this program contradict your physician's advice, be sure to consult your doctor before proceeding. Before starting any exercise program, always see your physician. The use of specific products in this book does not constitute an endorsement by the author or the publisher. The author and the publisher disclaim any liability or loss, personal or otherwise, resulting from the procedures in this program.

Mention of specific companies, organizations, or authorities in this book does not imply endorsement by the publisher, nor does mention of specific companies, organizations, or authorities in the book imply that they endorse the book.

Internet addresses and telephone numbers given in this book were accurate at the time the book went to press.

Printed in the United States of America

Rodale Inc. makes every effort to use acid-free ∞, recycled paper ♻.

Book design by Christopher Rhoads

Models: Andy McCutcheon and Angela Kenaston of Sports Unlimited

Library of Congress Cataloging-in-Publication Data

Darden, Ellington, date.
    The bowflex body plan : the power is yours : build more muscle : lose more fat / Ellington Darden.
        p.   cm.
    Includes bibliographical references and index.
    ISBN 1–57954–689–7 hardcover
    1. Exercise.   2. Bodybuilding—Training.
  3. Physical fitness.   I. Title.
    GV481.D34   2003
    613.7'1—dc21   2003011334

Distributed to the book trade by St. Martin's Press

4 6 8 10 9 7 5 3   hardcover

Visit us on the Web at www.rodalestore.com, or call us toll-free at (800) 848-4735.

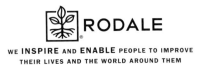

RODALE

WE INSPIRE AND ENABLE PEOPLE TO IMPROVE
THEIR LIVES AND THE WORLD AROUND THEM

ACKNOWLEDGMENTS

I acknowledge and thank the following people who made this project successful: Patty Moosbrugger for her agenting skills; Stephanie Tade for her publishing guidance; Troy Juliar for his editing; Jennifer Kushnier for her assistance; Jeanenne Darden for her creative advice; Mitch Mandel for his photography; Andy McCutcheon and Angela Kenaston for demonstrating the Bowflex exercises; Chris Rhoads for his layout and design; Randy Potter for his marketing ability; and Brian Cook for his overall support.

Special appreciation goes to all the men and women who participated in the research for this book, especially those whose pictures and stories are presented within.

CONTENTS

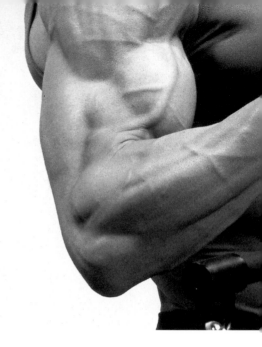

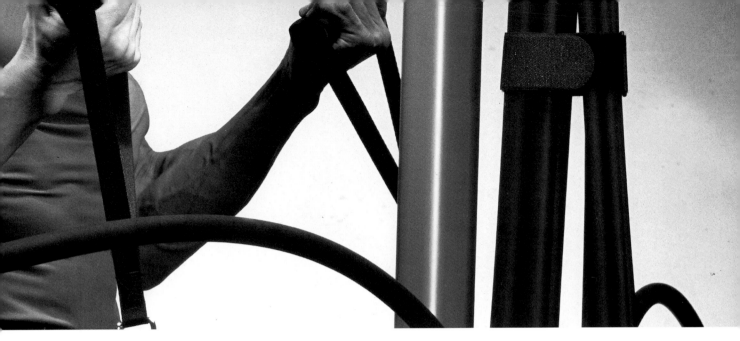

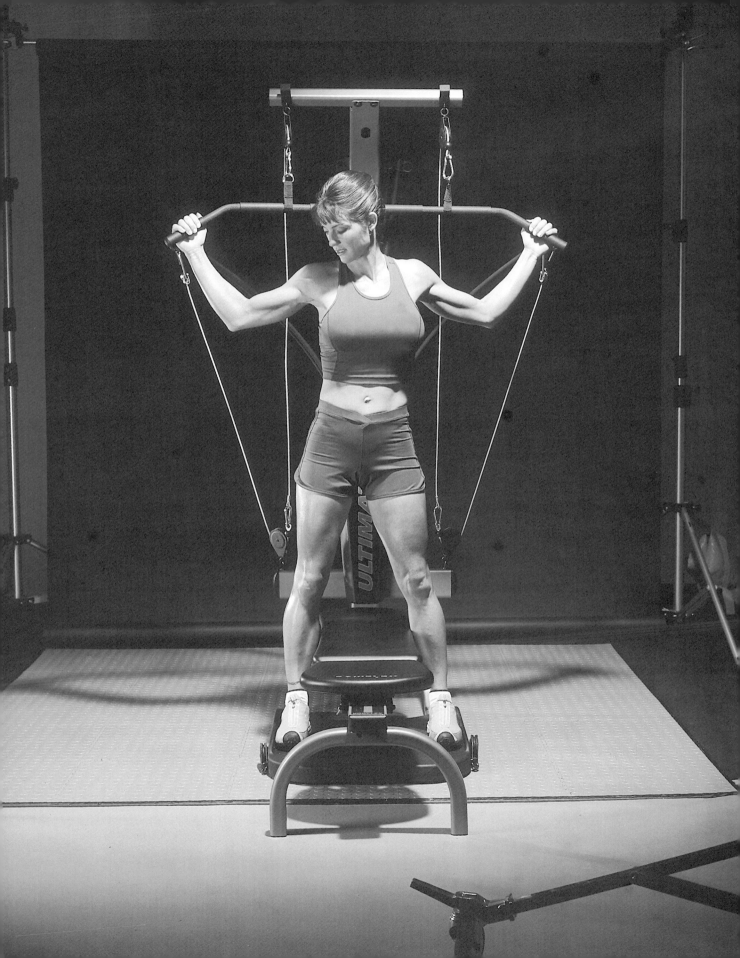

THE
BOWFLEX®
BODY PLAN

ACHIEVING A BOWFLEX BODY

The bending Power Rods supply resistance to Andy's clearly defined pectorals as his hands move across his torso.

As Angela's legs arc backward, shapely hamstrings show the effect of isolated leg curls.

With the Power Rods straightening, Andy's taut abdominals stretch and ready for another contraction.

Angela's legs extend against roller pads and her quadriceps separate into distinctive muscles that streamline her frontal thighs.

Andy's final repetition on the standing curl reveals a rounded biceps, whose strength perfectly matches the machine's force.

Andy McCutcheon, age thirty-six, and Angela Kenaston, age thirty-two, are pictured on the cover and throughout this book. Since 1999, they have been featured in many of the Bowflex television advertisements. Both Andy and Angela have trained intensely to build a Bowflex body.

A Bowflex body requires leanness and strength—a minimum of fat and above-average muscular development. Exercising, eating, hydrating, and resting—in precise amounts—are necessary to produce this look efficiently.

But let's face it. Not everyone has the genetics to look like Andy or Angela. Yet everyone can im-prove his or her body *significantly*. You don't have to resemble a cover model to achieve a Bowflex body. You just have to apply yourself as you eat smarter and train progressively on your Bowflex machine. With a little discipline and patience, you'll be amazed at the transformations that occur to your physique.

The book you're holding in your hands contains the best-possible, synergistic routines for building muscle and losing fat. Synergy occurs when the practices in this book interact to cause a greater effect than they would individually. This helps you create a leaner, stronger body *faster*. There are many different plans in this book. Choose one or more depending on your age, experience, body type, and goals. The emphasis in all the plans is always on effectiveness as opposed to novelty.

After only a short time of applying any of the plans, your excess fat will begin to disappear. You'll see your muscles' lean lines as well as subtle separations between body parts. You'll experience strength, firmness, and muscular refinement as never before.

Soon you'll have the results you've always wanted. Soon you'll have a Bowflex body.

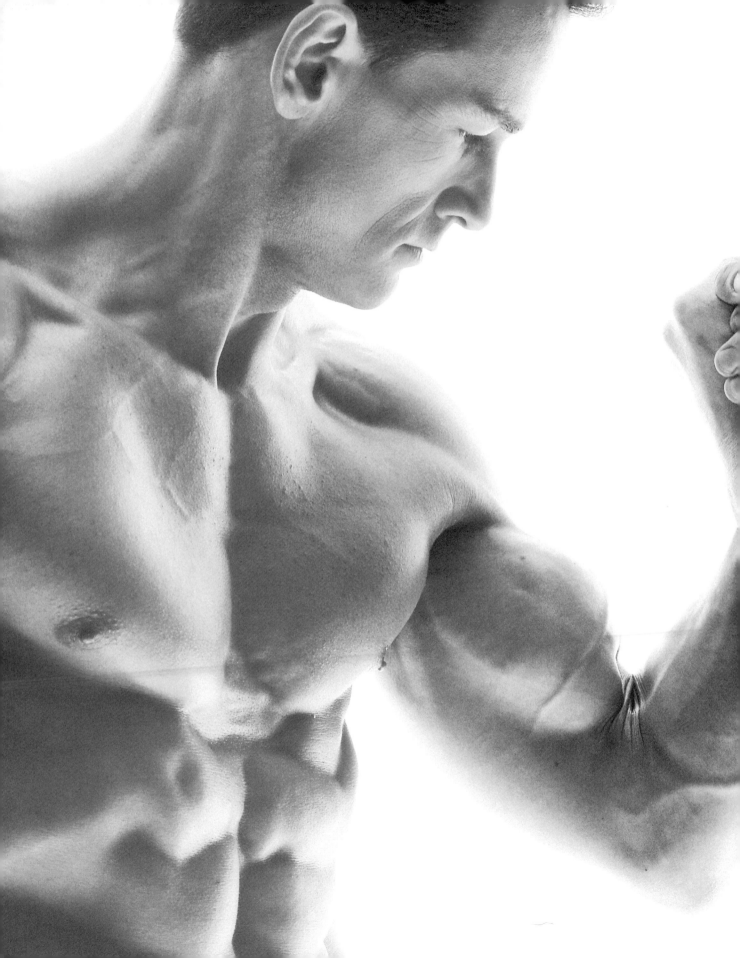

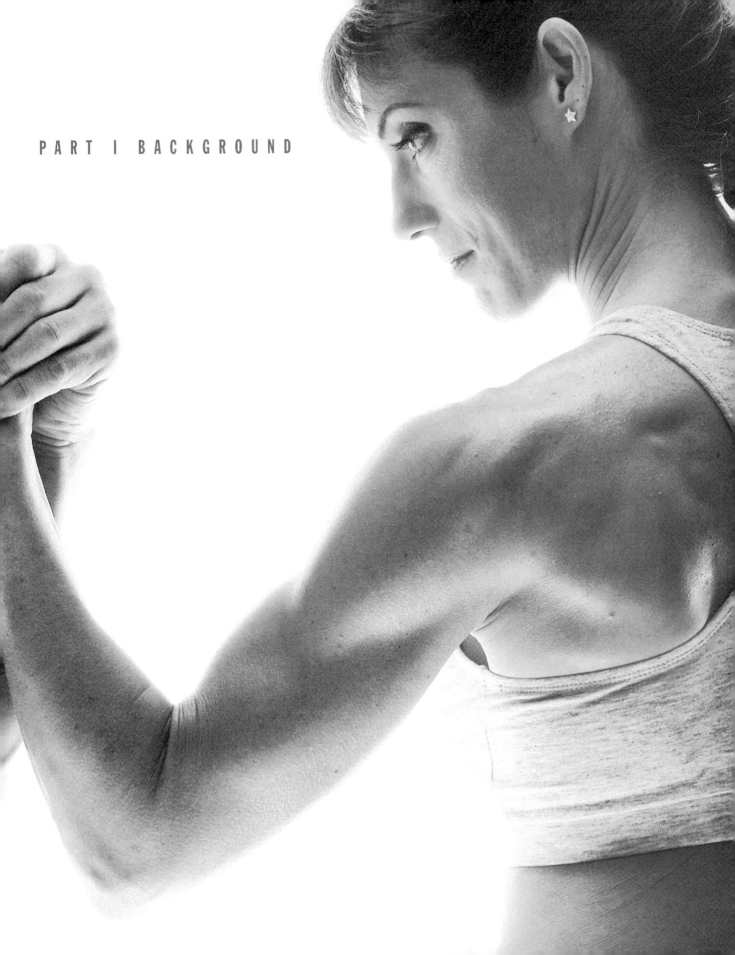

PART I BACKGROUND

1
THE POWER IS YOURS:

GET REAL RESULTS!

ONE OF THE MOST POPULAR TV commercials for Bowflex opens with a muscular man holding a bow, then pulling the string and arrow into a drawn position. The curve of the bow then transitions into a bending Power Rod on a Bowflex machine. The implication is that both bows provide force: the first to an arrow, the second to the human body.

The bow produces linear force and directs the arrow toward its target. The Power Rod bow exerts linear force, which is redirected through cables and pulleys to the targeted body part.

The bow and arrow revolutionized warfare for thousands of years because it was silent, lightweight, portable, and effective. Now, and because of the same reasons, the Bowflex exercise machine is revolutionizing home fitness.

That certainly wasn't the situation in December 1994, however, when I received a phone call from my friend, Dr. Wayne Westcott.

A CHALLENGE: "JUST TRY IT!"

"Bowflex? I'm not interested in testing any flimsy, unconventional home-exercise machine," I told Wayne, who was, and still is, the research director of the South Shore YMCA in Quincy, Massachusetts.

He's also the author of numerous books on strength training.

"But Ellington, we have a Bowflex machine in our facility," Westcott said, "and I believe you'll be surprised if you just try it." I pay attention when Westcott says something about strength training. But Bowflex? Well, I had to confront him on that.

At the time of our initial Bowflex discussion, I was living in Gainesville, Florida, where I was doing fat-loss research at the Gainesville Health and Fitness Center. Besides having more than 20,000 members, this fitness center has one of the largest arrays of strength-training equipment (Nautilus, MedX, Hammer, and free weights) in the United States. Everything here was heavy-duty. There were no home-exercise devices in sight!

I had seen a picture of a Bowflex machine in several magazines, but I had never actually tried one. Westcott, with his enthusiastic support, asked me to be open-minded about this particular home machine. Still, I was skeptical.

A month later, in January of 1995, Roland "Sandy" Wheeler, who at that time was vice president of marketing for Bowflex, visited me. Wheeler had located a man in Gainesville who owned a Bowflex machine and we were soon at that guy's home doing leg extensions, standing curls, and seated bench presses.

"Wow," I kept thinking to myself, "those leg extensions feel pretty good, and so do the standing curls. And the bench presses feel even better. But what about leg curls, leg presses, and pullovers? And let's not forget about abdominal crunches."

After another ten minutes of pushing, pulling, adjusting, and more pushing and pulling, I had my answers. Bowflex provided a nice resistance curve in most movements. It took only several seconds to change exercise positions. It was sturdy, but easy to move around. It certainly wasn't poorly designed, as I had initially imagined.

But how would it perform with test subjects who were used to heavy-duty equipment, and who wanted significant results?

A BOWFLEX STUDY

On the way back to the airport, I agreed with Wheeler that, indeed, Bowflex was worthy of a research study. Several weeks later, I had a Bowflex machine, which I stored in a closet on the second floor of the Gainesville Health and Fitness Center. I was ready to test if training on a Bowflex machine three times per week would build muscular size and strength to the same degree as free weights and heavy-duty exercise machines.

Strength training was not all I was concerned about. I was also interested in the connection between exercise and fat loss. Strength training, I've found, accelerates fat loss in three ways. First, it burns calories. Second, it elevates metabolic rate by rebuilding atrophied muscle or building new muscle. Third, it improves the body's shape and firmness, which in turn helps to keep the individual's motivation high.

My objective then, was to select, test, train, supervise, and retest a small group of overfat men and women on a six-week exercising and eating plan. The participants would train on Bowflex three times per week and adhere to a reduced-calorie diet each day. Body composition measurements would reveal the muscle gained and the fat lost.

SURPRISED? NO. OVERWHELMED? YES!

The research transpired without a hitch. I must confess, though, Westcott was wrong. I wasn't surprised by the Bowflex machine and the results of this six-week study. I was overwhelmed. Here's why.

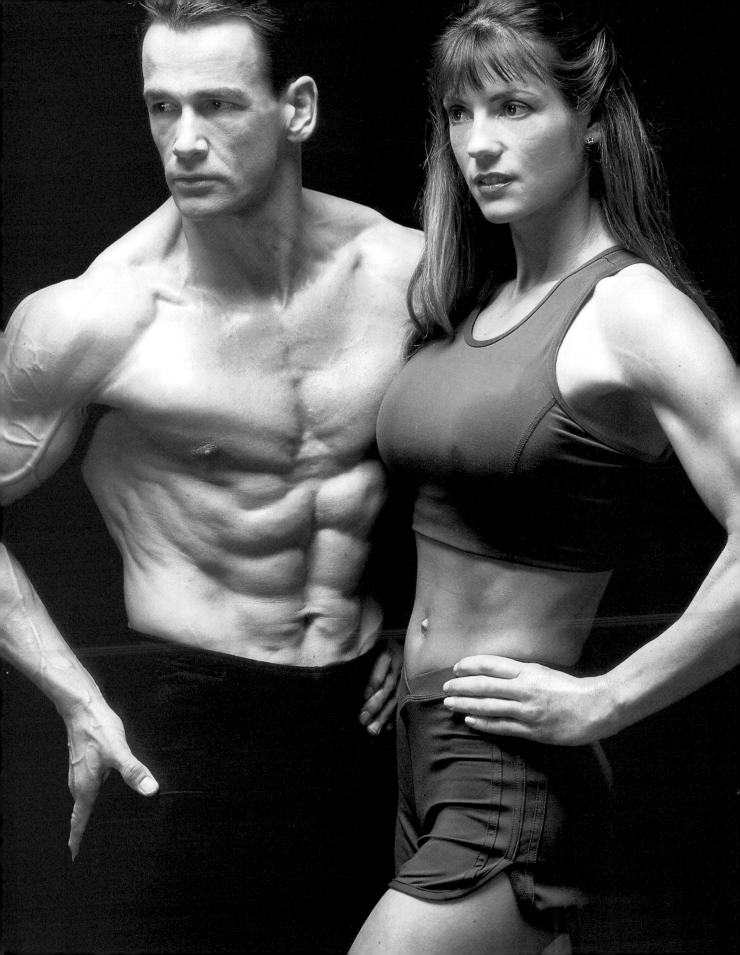

• Both the men and the women registered 100 percent compliance to the Bowflex workouts. In other words, no one missed a single one of the eighteen scheduled exercise sessions. I've never had 100 percent compliance in any of my previous studies. That says something about the ease of operation and the positive feedback the participants were receiving.

• The average muscle gained for each man was 3.7 pounds and the average gain per woman was 2.73 pounds. These figures are well within the range of gains for men and women whom I've trained with free weights and heavy-duty exercise machines. So, I concluded, Bowflex definitely stimulates muscular growth to a similar degree as does traditional strength-training equipment.

• Here's the real kicker: the average fat lost per man was 27.95 pounds and per woman was 16.96 pounds. Checking my records, before and after this six-week study, I've never had a group of men, nor women, perform better in overall fat loss. In fact, the Bowflex men established a new fat-loss record by 16 percent and the women did also by an even greater margin of 22.3 percent. Training on Bowflex seemed to keep the participants at a higher level of motiva-

tion. (Note: Just in case you might be curious about my experience, since 1966 I've personally supervised the exercising and eating of more than 10,000 individuals. Much of this research has been reported in my more than forty published books.)

You can read all about the particulars of the Bowflex research, and view the before-and-after photos, in chapter 20, The Body-Leanness Plan. I know now that one of the primary reasons that the Body-Leanness Plan produced such outstanding fat loss, even in the initial research stage, was synergy. For a complete discussion of synergy, see chapter 18.

In the fall of 1995, the Body-Leanness Plan was condensed and printed in the *Bowflex Owner's Manual and Fitness Guide*. Since then, thousands and thousands of Bowflex users have incorporated some, or all, of the program into their quest for strength and leanness.

THE EMERGENCE OF BOWFLEX

That fat-loss study was the beginning of a long association with Bowflex that continues to flourish. In 1996 I appeared in a successful Bowflex television infomercial, which is still being aired. Bowflex has gone from a seldom heard word to a concept that has grown to the most recognized name in home fitness.

Not a bad record for a machine that before 1994 I had never seen, nor tried, and couldn't take seriously. I even accused it of being "flimsy." Was I ever mistaken—until I *personally* tried it.

Since then, I've thoroughly examined the Bowflex machine from all angles. I've taken it apart and I've reassembled it, not once, but several times. It's made from high-quality materials throughout. It's a serious strength-training machine, which provides progressive-resistance exercise for all your major muscles.

COMPREHENSIVE HELP NEEDED

Bowflex exercise produces physiological changes in your body, usually in the form of more muscle and less fat. The degree of these changes, however, is dependent not only on the selection of the exercises but also on the frequency of workout, sleep, hydration, and nutrition, as well as a lot of little things such as stress, recovery ability, past injuries, outside activities, and lifestyle practices. Any one of these variables can mean the difference between losing ¼ pound of fat per week and 4 pounds of fat per week. Of course, it took me the better part of

thirty years to understand the interaction of these variables—and exactly how to manipulate them for the best possible, synergistic results.

I get dozens of e-mail questions each week through the Bowflex Web site (www.Bowflex.com) from trainees who need help reaching specific fat-loss and/or body-shaping goals. I supply them with brief, spot-on answers—and with little background as to the *why*. I'm told that's what works best on the Internet. Brief answers satisfy for a while, until the trainee hits another roadblock or perhaps misunderstands the original advice. Obviously, for better results, more assistance should be available.

The Bowflex Body Plan gives me the chance to provide the *why* behind much of my advice and, equally important, the opportunity to cover many topics at once. In summary, in this book you get the specifics and the generalities, the facts and the background, combined with numerous routines and programs.

DYNAMIC ACTION COURSES

The Bowflex Body Plan is the definitive and exclusively authorized resource on exercising and eating for the more than 1 million users of Bowflex equipment. Specifically, this book:

"A Huge Uplifting Experience"

Jeff Warren, a thirty-year-old health professional in a hospital at Battle Ground, Washington, was 5 feet 11 inches tall and weighed 210 pounds when he made up his mind to begin the Body-Leanness Plan. He wanted to lose fat and build muscle. He accomplished both.

"It seems like I've been heavy my whole life," Jeff said. "And I've never been good at sticking to something and following through. But I kept seeing that challenging Bowflex ad on TV. Finally, one morning, while looking in the mirror—and getting more and more disgusted at what I saw—I decided to order the Bowflex machine."

When the machine arrived, Jeff assembled it and started reading about the Body-Leanness Plan. The day before, he had been grocery shopping and stockpiled his typical selections of junk food—soft drinks, candy, cookies, chips, and beer. More determined than ever, he got rid of those diet-sabotaging foods and returned to the grocery store and bought all the recommended meal selections. That's discipline.

"After one week," Jeff recalled, "my weight started dropping—and dropping. I couldn't believe it. Sometimes I'd have to reweigh myself three or four times each morning just to be sure the scale was accurate."

After four months, Jeff reached his goal. He lost 40 pounds and reduced his waist by 7 inches, his hips by 2½ inches, and his thighs by 4 inches. He now weighs 170 pounds, and he says his muscles are "definitely larger and stronger" than before.

"The last four months have been a huge uplifting experience," Jeff concluded. "I feel great and never want to go back to where I was. My goal now is to maintain my current weight and build more muscle—with Bowflex."

• Explores the history of Bowflex, why and how it works

• Analyzes critically the role of proper exercise in fitness and health

• Explains the science of fat loss and strength training

• Details and illustrates how to get maximum effect from each recommended Bowflex exercise

• Yields practical guidelines on how to synergize exercising and eating

• Supplies proven courses for men who want bigger arms, broader shoulders, thicker chests, and ripped abdominals; and for women who desire tighter tummies, thinner hips and thighs, and generally stronger, leaner bodies

• Answers numerous questions on dieting, adaptations, advanced techniques, plateaus, and maintenance

• Inspires by sharing before-and-after stories and photographs of people who have successfully been through the various plans

The Bowflex Body Plan furnishes many synergistic routines. Some have a duration of two weeks, others six weeks. And there are dozens of individualized workouts—all of which help you build muscle and burn fat.

HOW ABOUT A DRILL PRESS?

Arthur Jones, the inventor of Nautilus equipment, had a profound influence on me and my understanding of strength training. I worked closely with Jones for more than thirty years. He once said, "People who buy drill presses don't really want drill presses. They want what the drill presses produce: *holes.*"

Jones then drew parallels between *drill presses* and *exercise machines*, between *holes* and *results.*

You bought this book, but you don't really want a book. You want *results*—results you hope to get from following the book's guidelines. You expect changes in your body. You want a smaller waist, a more mus-

cular torso, thinner thighs, and a host of other improved body parts.

Well, you've come to the right place if you want a better physique—a body with less fat, more muscle, and firmer parts.

Incidentally, the Bowflex Power Rod technology now appears in a machine called the Schwinn Comp,

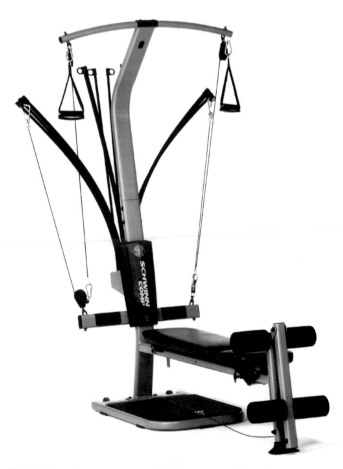

The Schwinn Comp is now available in stores nationwide.

available in many retail stores throughout the United States. Until now, Bowflex machines have been sold exclusively through television advertisements, 1-800 phone numbers, and Internet transactions. The instructions, guidelines, and programs in this book can be applied to all Bowflex machines, including the Schwinn Comp.

REAL PEOPLE, REAL RESULTS

Over the last several years, I've heard some remarkable stories from people who use Bowflex. I include them as sidebars throughout the book. As you read each story it might be helpful if you look for connections and similarities in your own life.

These stories are from men and women whose names have *not* been changed, who freely allowed me to use their actual names, city and state, measurements, interviews, and opinions. Unlike most fitness books, there are no composite people here.

These are real people—people just like you—who have jobs, spouses, kids, and day-to-day challenges and fitness problems. Each man and each woman took that first step, and then followed it with another, and another, and another.

MOTIVATION . . . DISCIPLINE . . . PATIENCE

Although all successful Bowflex users have a different story to tell, they have three things in common:

• *Motivation*—They are serious about changing their body.

• *Discipline*—They follow a plan of attack that usually includes an objective and a time frame.

• *Patience*—They endure the day-by-day, week-by-week, month-by-month regimen to reach their goal.

The Bowflex Body Plan educates and inspires in all three areas.

NOW, YOU'VE GOT THE POWER!

With this book and a Bowflex machine, *the power is yours* . . . to get the results you've always wanted.

Use the power.

Get real results.

2
FROM CREATION TO CREDIBILITY:

THE FACTS ABOUT
WHO, WHEN, & WHY

QUICK QUIZ—Who invented the Bowflex machine?

(a) Arthur Jones

(b) Vic Tanny

(c) Roland E. Wheeler

(d) Dosho Shifferaw

(e) Jack La Lanne

The answer to the above question is not classified by any means, but it certainly is not well known. First, the wrong choices.

Arthur Jones invented Nautilus and MedX equipment, but he didn't have a hand in the Bowflex machine. Vic Tanny was a famous gym owner in California, New York, and the Midwest in the 1950s and 1960s. Vic claimed that he invented the bench with racks to facilitate the barbell bench press, but he didn't have anything to do with Bowflex. Roland E. Wheeler is a longtime corporate director at Bowflex, but he didn't invent the machine. Jack La Lanne is a well-known fitness personality with no connections to Bowflex.

The correct answer is (d) Dosho Shifferaw. Yes, Shifferaw, a forty-seven-year-old entrepreneur now living in California, invented Bowflex. His story is fascinating.

A MAN FROM ETHIOPIA

Shifferaw was born in 1955 in Addis Ababa, Ethiopia. His father was in politics and eventually became a member of his country's parliament. When Dosho was twelve, his father bought him some dumbbells to help strengthen his body for sports. "I competed in soccer, basketball, and track and field," he remembered, "and the dumbbells helped me a lot."

He finished high school in Ethiopia in 1973 and, with his father's help, enrolled in Chapman College in Orange County, California, to study political science. Early the next year, tragedy struck. "All of a sudden," Shifferaw recalled, "there was a military revolution in Ethiopia. The communist rebels, in a matter of days, arrested my father, who was a senator in Emperor Haile Selassie's government, and killed him." The same thing happened to a lot of government officials. As a result, terrorism reigned in Ethiopia.

Shifferaw was devastated. Furthermore, his financial support from home was halted, so he dropped out of college. He made his way up the coast to San Francisco, where eventually he saved enough money from driving a taxi to continue his education. San Francisco City College provided him with a platform to study industrial design.

THE BREAKTHROUGH

During one of his industrial design classes, Shifferaw was behind schedule on a new prototype for a chair. As he was trying to decide what to do next, he casually placed a plastic rod across the back of his shoulders. As he walked around in deep thought, he naturally pulled a little on the ends of the rod. Then, he pulled harder. He looked at his arms and noticed that the muscles were contracting in bold relief.

"That's when the idea of getting resistance from bending a rod came to me," Shifferaw noted. "That led to a lot of learning about polymers and their properties."

It took a while, but Shifferaw finally built an effective prototype. "A friend was testing it," he continued, "and it looked just like a bow being pulled. I knew then that *Bowflex* was the natural name for the machine."

Shifferaw not only began refining his prototype, he took several classes in how to develop a business plan. At the same time, he worked on filing a patent. It took more than five years to get everything in order.

THE COOPERATIVE APPROACH

Shifferaw met Sandy Wheeler at a fitness convention in Lake Tahoe in 1984. Wheeler was interested in the machine and its unique way of providing resistance. Wheeler, in turn, got Brian Cook involved. Cook and Wheeler had been CPAs together in a large accounting firm in Seattle. They were both looking for products to manufacture and market.

In early 1985, Shifferaw incorporated Bowflex of America. Several months later, Wheeler and Cook successfully negotiated with him for a license of the Bowflex technology and then purchased a majority interest in the new company. The first Bowflex machine for the home was manufactured and sold in 1986.

"I have great respect for Brian Cook and Sandy Wheeler," Shifferaw said recently. "They made it happen."

THE MAGIC OF TEAMWORK

Success, however, didn't come quickly—nor easily. "I can remember displaying a Bowflex machine at some of the fitness conventions in 1987 and 1988," Cook noted, "and not a person walked into the booth. Not one single person tried the machine!" The concept of bending bows supplying resistance was not catching on among fitness professionals. A brief entry into the retail market looked promising, but after five years it didn't pan out.

Randy Potter joined the team in 1991 as creative director and marketing manager. Randy updated the Bowflex literature and concentrated on making videotapes about Bowflex. The videotapes were both instructional and educational. Then, the next part of Potter's job began—to aggressively expand Bowflex's television marketing. In 1993, direct marketing became a focal point for the company.

At the same time, several improvements were made to the machine's design. The seat, for example, had always rested on the floor. It was raised to 14 inches. Tom Purvis, a registered physical therapist from Oklahoma City, was consulted in 1995 and provided valuable suggestions involving biomechanics and efficiency. Attachments were developed. Eventually, three different Bowflex machines and eight different models were offered.

The modifications to the machine and the marketing creativity got attention. People began to take notice, try the machine, and *like the feel.* Sales picked up significantly in 1996 and 1997.

In 1998, the direct marketing of Bowflex through cable television advertisements and 1-800 call centers began to produce significant sales. The concept was earning credibility. Bowflex was now on its way to becoming a high-visibility product.

Brian Cook, chairman, has an overriding philosophy that he strongly believes in, which is a fitting close to this section on the Bowflex history. He says, "Success is produced not by any individual but, rather, by a *team* of people." And then he follows up with, "When you think you're doing good— that's when you'd better watch out. Stay humble and stay focused."

BOWFLEX TECHNOLOGY

In simple terms, Bowflex works because, as Dosho Shifferaw noticed in 1979, a polymer rod has the potential to provide resistance. Bend it with your arms and you can feel your muscles contracting.

The key, however, was a combination of perfecting the polymer and then learning how to harness the resistance efficiently. That's what Bowflex has accomplished with precision. A brief description of the major components of a Bowflex machine reveals how this precision is accomplished.

Power Rods. It all begins with the Power Rod resistance technology. Each rod is composed of solid polymer material called Poly-Hexamethaline-Adipamide, which is sheathed in protective black rubber coating. The rods are 4 feet long and are

"I Now Have to Buy My Pants from the Junior Section"

Diane Tatters, age forty-three, is a purchasing agent and mother of two grown children in Trafford, Pennsylvania. Over the years, the stress of her job, combined with poor eating and exercising habits, had allowed her body weight to balloon to 180 pounds—which is a lot for a woman only 5 feet 2 inches tall.

"For many years," Diane remembered, "my husband and I would purchase gym memberships and be gung ho about losing weight. After about a month, we'd find excuses and that was the end of that—until the next year, when we'd repeat the process again. We've donated a lot of money to the local fitness center."

Enter the Bowflex Power Pro into the life of the Tatterses in July 2000.

"My husband and I both like to work out in the early morning," Diane continued. "That compact little Bowflex machine makes exercise so convenient for us. I never miss a workout, not even when I'm rushed."

The discipline of not missing a single workout and sticking to a lower-calorie diet certainly paid big dividends for Diane. After eight months, she had shed 65 pounds. Her clothes went from a size 16 to a size 3 to 5.

"In fact, I now have to buy my pants from the junior section," she beamed. "I feel better at age forty-three than I did at thirty. And get this: my husband now holds my hand when we're out on the town—which makes me feel real good. Of course, he's lost 70 pounds himself by following the Bowflex program, which makes me want to hold his hand, too.

"Best of all, I've kept my weight off for more than a year now. Bowflex has changed my life for the better and I'm so thankful."

manufactured in four different diameters. The thicker the rod, the more resistance it provides. The resistance, which is marked on the rod cap, begins at 5 pounds and ends with 50 pounds. The Bowflex Ultimate, for example, comes with one pair of 5-pound rods, two pairs of 10-pound rods, one pair of 30-pound rods, and two pairs of 50-pound rods. The lightest resistance you can hook onto the machine is

5 pounds. The heaviest, with upgrades, is 410 pounds. Endurance testing on the rods revealed that it took more than 1 million bends or flexes before any significant weakening occurred.

Bowflex stands strongly behind its patented Power Rod technology. If there are any problems or failures, before or after a million repetitions, Bowflex will replace the rod at no charge.

Frame. The frame of the machine has to be strong and durable to anchor the Power Rod technology and to support an exercising individual, especially a large person who weighs more than 250 pounds. The tubular steel frame is heavy gauge and protected with a powder-coated, oven-baked finish.

Seat, bench, and platform. The Bowflex machine has four basic bench positions: flat, incline, free sliding, and totally removed. Each position is governed by adjustments of the spring lock pin on the side of the seat. Both the bench and seat are made of polyurethane, not vinyl-covered foam. The bottom platform is constructed of high-density, molded plastic.

Cables and pulleys. The cables are composed of aircraft-grade steel with a 2,000-pound tensile strength rating and are covered with a protective nylon jacket. Nylon coating lasts much longer than vinyl, which tends to crack. The side pulleys and various attachment pulleys are custom-made with sealed bearings. They are designed for quiet, smooth, long-term operation.

Hand grips/ankle cuffs. Bowflex even has patented handles that work three ways—as regular grips, as no-grip handcuffs, and as ankle harnesses. The handles are easy to adjust and provide safety and confidence when performing the various exercises.

Attachments. Bowflex manufactures several accessories and attachments that fit the standard machine. There's a long bar for barbell-type exercises and a short T-bar for concentrated arm and back work. For working the hips and thighs there's a squat-bar attachment. For pulldowns and triceps pushdowns, Bowflex has a lat-tower addition. The leg-extension/leg-curl attachment focuses on strengthening the quadriceps and hamstrings.

YOUR WEAPON OF CHOICE

Combine the correct components—Power Rods, frame, seat, bench, platform, cables, pulleys, hand grips, and attachments—and you have a machine that furnishes lineal progressive resistance in both concentric and eccentric phases. You have a machine that delivers an excellent range of motion for more than sixty strength-building exercises.

Consider a Power Rod and an archer's bow. Both tools provide force. Both supply resistance. Both are precision, result-producing weapons. Bowflex is now your weapon of choice—*your weapon of choice in the fight for strength and leanness.*

3

THE COMPONENTS OF A FIT BODY:

ENDURANCE, FLEXIBILITY, STRENGTH, & LEANNESS— WHICH IS THE MOST IMPORTANT?

"IF I COULD DO ONLY ONE FORM of training from now on, I'd give up cardio and focus on strength training."

That quote sounds like something you'd hear from Arnold Schwarzenegger, doesn't it? Well, it's not. It's from Kathy Smith, who has produced twenty-six cardio-aerobic videos that have sold more than 11 million copies.

I first met Kathy in 1978 when she visited the Nautilus headquarters. Even then, I was impressed with her knowledge of strength training and her motivation to work intensely. At that time, Kathy Smith had one of the best-built bodies I'd ever seen.

I also talked with Arnold Schwarzenegger several times in the 1970s when he was a champion bodybuilder, and later worked with him when he headed the President's Council on Physical Fitness. Up close, he's very personable and nearly bigger-than-life, with his large, muscular physique. He, too, had one of the best bodies ever.

Today, Kathy and Arnold, each over fifty years of age, are both devoted to strength training—and they still have great bodies. Arnold and Kathy realized early that the most important factor in getting the body you want is building muscle mass. Kathy explains this clearly in her book, *Lift Weights to Lose Weight*, which was published in 2001. Although Smith's book is pri-marily directed to women, men also follow a similar pattern of gradually losing muscle as they age.

As people get older, this wasting away of muscle sets off a chain reaction, leading to a loss of strength, a reduction of bone density, a drop in metabolic rate, and an increase in fat. None of the above helps you look better.

Muscle gives your body support, contour, and firmness. Without it, you'd be a stick person with globs of fat causing unsightly protrusions.

The solution is to prevent the loss of muscle mass, or even increase it. And there is no better way to increase your muscle mass than with strength training.

COMPONENTS OF PHYSICAL FITNESS

Strength training deals with more than your muscles, or at least it should. That's why it's important to understand the major components of a fit body. It's generally agreed that physical fitness is composed of four factors: cardiovascular endurance, joint flexibility, muscular strength, and body leanness. Let's briefly examine each one.

Cardiovascular endurance. The cardiovascular system consists of the heart, arteries, capillaries, and veins. The heart is a muscle that serves as both a storage tank and a pump for moving blood through the body. Arteries are tubular vessels that carry blood away from the heart. Capillaries are tiny single-layer vessels in the tissues themselves where the actual exchange of oxygen, nutrients, and waste materials takes place. The capillaries then connect with a system of small, then larger veins that return the blood to the heart for recirculation.

Obviously, a fit individual needs to be able to pump blood to and from the working muscles effectively and efficiently. If not, then performance suffers.

To improve the endurance of the cardiovascular system, three criteria must be met. One, the exercise must be hard enough to get the heart rate up to 70 to 85 percent of its maximum beats per minute. Two, this elevated heart rate must be sustained for a minimum of 10 minutes. Three, such exercise should be repeated at least three times per week.

Joint flexibility. Flexibility is the range of movement around a joint. Increase the range of movement and you may be able to generate more force in a given activity.

Stretching is the key to increasing flexibility. An individual must be pushed or pulled into a stretched position that temporarily exceeds his existing range of movement. For best results, all stretching should be done slowly and smoothly.

Muscular strength. Strength is the ability of the muscles to exert force. From blinking the eyes and wiggling the nose to vigorous running and throwing—muscles, by contracting and relaxing, make all human movements possible. Overloading the muscles in a progressive manner is what makes them stronger.

The size and strength of the muscles is a major factor in determining how your body looks. More muscle means better body contours, not only for men but especially for women.

Besides movement and shape, high levels of muscular strength can prevent injuries. In most cases, excessive force causes injury. When a force exceeds the structural integrity of the human body, injury is the result. Everyone should increase the structural integrity of his or her body. Stronger muscles equal stronger bodies. Strength training allows not only the muscles to grow stronger but also the tendons, ligaments, connective tissues, and even the bones.

Body leanness. Leanness is the opposite of fatness. Excessive fat on the body does not contribute to movement, performance, or health. Leanness is best produced by simultaneously losing fat and building muscle.

TRADITIONAL EXERCISE PROGRAMS

Tradition in exercise may be good because it keeps people grounded. Or tradition in exercise may be bad, if it prevents people from applying something different.

Many fitness-minded people—in spite of research to the contrary—continue to have separate routines for cardiovascular endurance, joint flexibility, and muscular strength. For example, a man might jog three miles for cardiovascular endurance, do calisthenic-type stretching for flexibility, and lift barbells for strength. A woman, typically, might do an aerobics class for cardio, yoga for flexibility, and a dumbbell routine for strength.

Each one of these activities would require a minimum of 30 minutes and each would be repeated three times per week. Adding that up, it's 90 minutes times three, or 270 minutes (4½ hours) per week devoted to exercise.

Four and a half hours a week doesn't sound like a lot of time, so that shouldn't be a problem, right? Wrong. According to a survey done by the International Health, Racquet and Sportsclub Association (IHRSA), "not having enough time," is one of the leading reasons why people don't exercise.

What if that time, however, could be reduced from 4½ hours a week to 1½ hours a week? Maybe you can't spare 90 minutes a day, but how about 30 minutes?

The secret to paring all those separate routines down to 30 minutes is strength training—strength training that is organized and performed in the correct manner. To appreciate this concept, you may need help with some old stereotypes.

CHIPPING AWAY AT STEREOTYPES

When I was in graduate school at Florida State University in 1969, I was a subject in a study that involved performing a circuit of barbell exercises. My heart rate and oxygen consumption were monitored throughout the workout. Not surprising to me, I found that both my heart rate and oxygen consumption were in the range necessary for cardiovascular conditioning. The key factor in this was rapidly moving from one exercise to another—within 15 to 30 seconds. To accomplish this, all the weights had to be set beforehand.

This study, which was part of an unpublished master's thesis, went against the grain of what was believed at that time. In 1968, Dr. Kenneth Cooper had published *Aerobics* and it pushed the concept of long, enduring, low-intensity exercise for benefiting the cardiovascular system. Cooper, in his book, evaluated

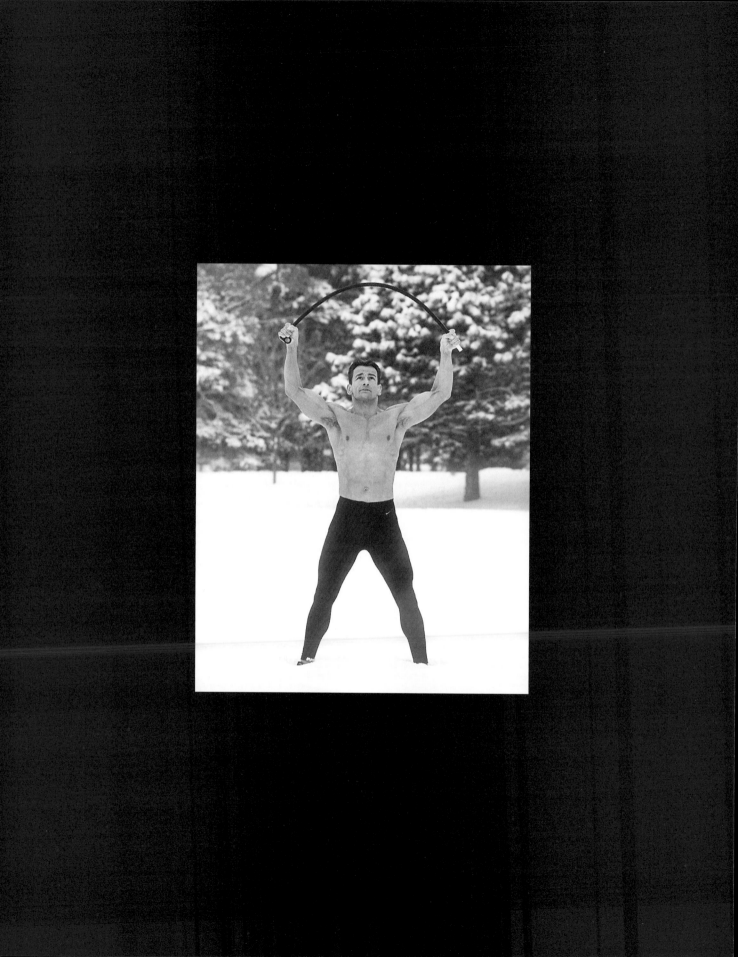

and ranked various activities. Cross-country skiing, swimming, and jogging were at the top, followed by cycling and walking. Strength training was ranked near the bottom, along with golf, shuffleboard, and bowling.

The reason strength training ranked so low had to do with the way the tested participants exercised. In the 1960s, people who strength-trained were called weight lifters and bodybuilders. *Strength training* as a conditioning approach didn't become popular until ten years later. Anyway, the weight lifters and bodybuilders who Cooper tested were trained in the traditional manner: 15 seconds or less of explosive-type lifting followed by a several-minute rest period. They would continue these lifting-resting cycles for an hour or more.

It should be obvious that these weight lifters and bodybuilders, who trained in the traditional manner, were not elevating their heart rates long enough for cardiovascular conditioning to occur. Naturally, they performed poorly on endurance-type tests. There were plenty of athletes in the 1960s who strength-trained with higher repetitions and briefer rest periods, but they weren't selected for Cooper's study.

Thus, a stereotype—that weight lifting provided poor aerobic or cardiovascular conditioning—was established in 1968. To make matters worse, this new stereotype joined hands with a fifty-year-old stereo-type, that weight lifting makes a person muscle-bound and inflexible.

Both assumptions were incorrect, then as well as now.

THE BEGINNING OF A REVOLUTION

When I joined Arthur Jones and his Nautilus Sports/Medical Industries in 1973, I was impressed that Jones wanted not only to better understand a barbell but also to improve its function. The end result was a Nautilus exercise machine for almost every major muscle group of the body.

These machines were unlike anything the exercise world had seen before. They were large, tubular-steel, open devices with chains, redirectional pulleys, odd-shaped cams, movement arms, seats, belts, and weight stacks, which altogether worked amazingly well. By organizing ten to twelve Nautilus machines around a room, and ordering the machines according to the size of the muscle group (from larger to smaller), a trainee could perform a complete circuit in 20 to 30 minutes.

Nautilus, in only a few years, brought weight lifting and bodybuilding out of the dark ages and introduced the new concept of *strength training* to the masses.

More important, Nautilus made strength training inviting and accessible.

One of the first projects that we undertook at Nautilus was to study the fitness parameters of motivated individuals using Nautilus equipment. The United States Military Academy at West Point, New York, with its corps of cadets, contained the ideal individuals. Subsequently, Nautilus and the Military Academy organized a joint project under the direction of Dr. James A. Peterson. In 1975, I helped circuit-train twenty cadets, who were varsity football players, for six weeks.

In only seventeen workouts averaging fewer than 30 minutes each, these athletes increased their strength an average of 59 percent in each of ten exercises. They improved their flexibility by 7.22 inches in trunk extension and 5.5 inches in shoulder flexion. They improved their cardiovascular endurance so much that they reduced their times for the two-mile run by 88 seconds.

The stereotype that strength training doesn't improve cardiovascular endurance or increase flexibility did not hold true at the Military Academy.

I was at West Point for the duration of this study and was amazed at the motivation of these student athletes. Their achievements were real and hard-earned. Since this was a Nautilus-funded project and the results challenged several mainstream beliefs, some critics questioned the validity of the study, especially as to how it related to cardiovascular conditioning.

SETTLING THE ISSUE

In 1985, Dr. Stephen Messier and Mary Dill of Wake Forest University helped to settle the issue by publishing a study in the *Research Quarterly for Exercise and Sport*. They measured the aerobic conditioning benefits of thirty-six male college students divided into three groups: (1) those training on Nautilus equipment, (2) those lifting free weights in the traditional style, and (3) those engaged in a running program. All subjects trained three times per week for ten weeks.

The findings showed the Nautilus trainees enjoyed the same aerobic benefits that the runners did. Furthermore, the running group trained 50 percent longer than the Nautilus group—30 minutes per session compared to 20 minutes per session. The group that exercised in the traditional lifting fashion actually performed slightly worse in the cardiovascular tests at the end than at the beginning.

Soon several more studies, published in well-known journals, revealed similar results. The exercise-physiology world was finally seeing what numerous fitness enthusiasts had been experiencing for fifteen years.

"Where Do You Work Out?"

"I'm interested in muscular development," noted forty-one-year-old Adam Brooks, who is a state game and fish employee in Helena, Montana. "For most of my life, I was one of those tall guys—skinny everywhere except my waist—with no chest muscles and thin arms. I hated to be seen in shorts or without a shirt. I tried a few popular bodybuilding programs, but I ended up getting hurt."

After a painful divorce in early 2000, Adam's body weight skyrocketed to 275 pounds. "I sort of let myself go," he recalled. But at a height of 6 feet 4 inches, Adam was still skinny, even though his belly was huge. "A Bowflex, with all the upgrades, was the very first purchase I made after moving into my own place." The date was July 2, 2000.

Adam began with the Body-Leanness Plan, with one addition. Because of his overall size and height, plus having an active, outdoor job, he added 500 calories to the basic 1,500-calorie-a-day diet. He worked out every other day on the bodybuilding routine recommended in the *Bowflex Owner's Manual*.

The results were quick. By the end of August, Adam had lost 55 pounds and was down to 221 pounds. His waistline had shrunk by 7 inches. Six months later, Adam figured his muscle mass had increased by at least 7 pounds because he had added 2 inches to his biceps and 4 inches on his chest.

"Now, my waist is virtually flat, my arms are much bigger, and my chest actually sticks out farther than my gut for the first time in my life," Adam noted. "Often when I meet people who don't know me, they ask, 'Where do you work out?' or even better, 'How long have you been bodybuilding?'

"For someone like me, who has been so skinny for so long, that's absolutely the best."

Strength training, properly performed with only brief rest periods between exercises, can significantly increase your cardiovascular endurance.

Strength training will also, if attention is given to stretching in appropriate positions, make you more flexible. And strength training will, of course, increase your muscular strength.

Nautilus started a revolution in strength training by establishing the philosophy that you could get high levels of cardiovascular endurance, joint flexibility, and muscular strength from a single, brief exercise session that is repeated three times per week. Ninety minutes a week versus 270 minutes a week—*the same or better results in one-third the time!*

From 1980 through 1998, I expanded that philosophy with my fat-loss studies and publications. For example, *The Nautilus Diet* (1987), *The Six-Week Fat-to-Muscle Makeover* (1988), *32 Days to a 32-Inch Waist* (1990), *Hot Hips and Fabulous Thighs* (1991), and *A Flat Stomach ASAP* (1998) all proved that strength training combined with a reduced-calorie diet produced maximum fat loss and body leanness.

COMPARING THE OTHER COMPONENTS

Cardiovascular endurance, joint flexibility, muscular strength, and body leanness, as I've mentioned, are the four components of physical fitness, and research reveals that strength training has positive effects on all four components. But what about working one of the other factors exclusively? Will doing so produce benefits in any of the other three?

I've seen long-distance runners who exercised their cardiovascular systems exclusively, sometimes for years and years. Such running, no doubt, significantly improves cardiovascular endurance. Because running is a repetitive, mid-range movement, no end-of-motion stretching is involved. So running does not increase joint flexibility. Long-distance running, by the very nature of the activity, is not intense enough to stimulate the major muscles of the body to grow

stronger, at least not past a certain low level. In fact, some runners actually overtrain their legs to the point that their muscles atrophy. Running does little or nothing for muscular strength. But running, because it burns calories (the number burned is dependent on age, body weight, skill, intensity, and duration), can certainly contribute to leanness.

In the final analysis, running to improve cardiovascular endurance can have a positive effect on body leanness but poor or no effect on joint flexibility and muscular strength.

Most other cardio activities such as aerobic routines that involve dancing and stepping, cycling, spinning, swimming, walking, and using a treadmill will also have little or no effect on flexibility or strength. They do, however, effectively work the cardiovascular system and contribute to body leanness.

What about those who participate in stretching movements, such as yoga and Pilates? They concentrate on increasing joint flexibility through slow movements and focused breathing. They are rewarded with additional flexibility, but little improvement in the other three components of fitness.

Finally, will concentrating on body leanness through reduced-calorie dieting help endurance, flexibility, or strength? Perhaps to a degree, especially if a person is obese. Losing significant fat pounds and inches will improve the function of the heart and probably increase the flexibility of some joints. During muscular contraction, fat between muscle fibers acts as a friction brake, so shrinking fat cells could lead to better movement.

On the other hand, dieting without strength training causes an indiscriminant loss of weight, some of which comes from the muscles. Such reduction of muscle mass is not desirable because it makes a person weaker and lowers his or her metabolic rate. Thus, focusing on dieting alone for leanness is not recommended.

Before getting back to the efficiency of strength training, it should be recognized that some individuals strength train only for weight lifting, powerlifting, or bodybuilding purposes. They may not care about cardiovascular endurance or joint flexibility, and consequently they get very little of either from their workout. Strength training must be understood and properly applied for maximum benefits to occur across all four areas of fitness.

KATHY AND ARNOLD ARE RIGHT

If you could do only one form of training from now on, what would it be?

Kathy Smith is right. And so are Arnold Schwarzenegger, The Rock, Cory Everson, Kiana Tom, and thousands of others who have experienced significant results from lifting weights. Strength training produces maximum results with minimum investment of time.

But what kind of equipment do Smith and Schwarzenegger use? According to their most recent books, they use a combination of free weights and machines. Nothing was mentioned about Bowflex. But that's not important—*really!* What matters is that strength training is an integral part of their weekly lifestyles.

Regardless of the strength-training tool—Bowflex, Nautilus, MedX, Cybex, Hammer, free weights, or other types—the most important factor is *how you apply whatever equipment you have.* Use it correctly and you'll get stronger, fitter, and leaner.

Strength training is the most important factor in physical fitness.

Strength training—compared to running, cycling, swimming, cardio-aerobic classes, yoga, and Pilates—is efficiency in action. Strength training is the best way to achieve the body you want.

The next chapter zeros in on strength training at home and why Bowflex offers so much convenience.

4

THE GYM EXPLOSION:

THERE'S NO PLACE LIKE HOME

IN 1959, WHEN I FIRST BECAME interested in strength training, there was no commercial gym in my hometown of Conroe, Texas. Conroe, with a population of 10,000, is located forty miles north of Houston. Like some people of that day, I purchased a barbell-dumbbell set from my local sporting goods store and trained with it in my parents' garage.

Today that has changed. There's probably a commercial gym or a not-for-profit fitness facility (YMCA, corporate, municipal, hospital, university, high school, or military) that is within driving distance from where you live or work. In 1959 there were fewer than 2,000 such workout places throughout the United States. In 2002, according to the International Health, Racquet and Sportsclub Association, the commercial clubs and the not-for-profit facilities together totaled more than 37,000.

These 37,000 clubs and facilities have approximately 34 million members. Interestingly, IHRSA's 1999 report, *50 Million Members by 2010*, pointed out that 90 percent of health clubs lose from 30 to 50 percent of their total membership each year. In fact, almost anywhere you visit in the United States, there are twice as many former members of gyms as there are current members, which is an amazing statistic.

WHY PEOPLE QUIT

Surveys by the IHRSA indicate that most people drop their memberships due to this primary reason:

• They don't use the facility enough to justify the cost. In other words, they can't find the time to make it consistently to the gym.

This was followed closely by a number of anxieties, namely the fear of feeling:

• Stupid because of ignorance of how the club or equipment works

• Athletically incompetent relative to more experienced members

• Socially isolated in an arena that is inherently social and interactive

• That their physique is inferior and out of shape

Finally, there were several more reasons why people quit:

• Overcrowded facilities

• Unresponsive staff

• Dissatisfaction with programs

IHRSA, with its goal of 50 million members by 2010, has a tough road ahead—especially if you're talking about satisfied members who are getting results.

WELCOME HOME, ENTER BOWFLEX

Surveys show that, compared to joining a gym, twice as many people choose to exercise at home. That's a total of 74 million people. These individuals are combating some of the reasons used to drop out of fitness centers—you don't have to worry about being a klutz, feeling stupid, looking out of shape, or not wearing the right attire. The staff and management at home should also be more to your liking!

Then, there's the number one reason people quit: people sign up for gym memberships with good intentions, but after the novelty wears off they seldom go.

Why? Because it takes time. Perhaps an hour and a half or even two hours of time is required to drive to the gym, find a parking place, dress, wait for the equipment, do the exercises, shower, redress, and drive home. Now, repeat those procedures three days per week, consistently!

With a Bowflex machine at home, the time issue becomes minimal. There's no drive time, no trouble finding a place to park, no wait for the equipment, and your Bowflex is always ready for business.

When it's at your home, you'll probably use it more than you think. With the instructions and programs in this book, I'm sure you will.

MY HOME GYM NOW

At one time I strength-trained in my garage with barbells and dumbbells. Today, my training environment has expanded—considerably.

I live and work in a home that my wife and I built in 2000. My wife, Jeanenne, is an interior designer in Orlando. In the east wing of our home, overlooking a lake, we have a gym—a gym that Jeanenne customized for me. It consists of a 14-foot arched ceiling, supported by three massive, black wooden beams. The floor is wide-planked yellow pine that is distressed and stained black. The end wall is old-style brick with weeping mortar. The other walls and ceiling are beige. It's a great atmosphere that is very conducive to exercise.

What kind of equipment do I have in my gym? The centerpiece is a Bowflex Ultimate machine. Along with the Bowflex, I have five Nautilus machines. From this equipment, I have created several routines that I alternate using. Approximately 60 percent of the exercises I do are performed on the Bowflex machine.

Since I've had my new home gym, I haven't exercised in a commercial fitness center. Everything I require for a complete workout is now in my home.

Toned, Confident, and Looking Good

Karen Dougher, forty-five, is married and the mother of two boys. She resides in Liverpool, New York, where she is an executive administrative assistant. She bought her Bowflex Power Pro in May of 2001. At 5 feet 5 inches tall and with a weight of 143 pounds, Karen simply wanted to tone her muscles.

"I work at a pretty stressful job," Karen explained, "so I need to relax when I get home after work. To help me do this, I set up the Bowflex machine in an extra bedroom upstairs. There's a lot of sunlight up there and also a stereo. I like to put on George Winston's piano music while exercising. Both the music and the Bowflex, at a smooth pace, help to calm me down. After an hour of this, I feel relaxed and invigorated—both mentally and physically."

It took only six weeks of this three-times-per-week exercising and relaxing for her body to respond. With little or no changes in her diet (she has been practicing low-fat eating for at least seven years), Karen dropped 8 pounds of fat and added 3 to 5 pounds of body-defining muscle.

"I'm probably in the best shape I've been in twenty years, since before I had my kids," Karen commented. "My arms are very muscular and toned, my calves are rock hard, and my stomach is nice and sculpted.

"My husband is thrilled with the way my body looks now. He comments every day on how my hips and butt have decreased and how my chest is so toned. I was able to get back into my size-8 jeans—and they are actually too loose now. All my friends from bowling and softball have told me how great I look. It really is a self-confidence booster to know you look good to others.

"Most of all, however, I look good to me. Thanks, Bowflex."

What's best for me, however, may or may not be best for you.

YOUR HOME GYM

Most people don't have the room to house the various machines that I do. Nor do they want to spend the money on all the equipment. They do, however, have the finances to buy a Bowflex machine and enough space to use it. The innovative design of Bowflex allows it to fold quickly into a compact unit and roll into or out of a closet or storage area.

Your Bowflex machine may be set up in almost any room in your home. It does make sense, however, to use it in an area that is conducive to serious training. The ideal room would be fairly open, well-ventilated, cool, quiet, and off-limits to young children. Of course, you can make do in tight quarters, in an attic, and even in a garage if necessary.

One buddy of mine, who is on the road six months out of the year, carries his Bowflex with him inside his recreational vehicle. When the weather is nice, he often stops, sets his Bowflex up in a nice park, and trains outdoors.

Don't let the lack of an ideal space deter you from using your Bowflex machine. Start now. You can get more creative with your training room after the first several weeks of the program.

BOWFLEX AND COMMERCIAL FITNESS

What about a series of Bowflex machines being used in a commercial fitness center? There's been some interest in this concept, but even the Bowflex Ultimate, with its larger-gauge tubular steel, is not designed to be placed on the floor of a gym where it would be subjected to constant use, and possibly abuse, by hundreds of people weekly.

In 1999, Direct Focus, the parent company of Bowflex, acquired Nautilus strength-training equipment and its powerful brand. In 2002, Direct Focus was renamed The Nautilus Group. Today, the concept of a cable system with sealed-bearing pulleys that swivel and adapt, which Bowflex uses so successfully, has been similarly applied to various Nautilus multistation machines. These multistation machines have weight stacks, instead of Power Rods, and are being marketed to commercial fitness centers. In a club setting, it is the closest equipment there is to a Bowflex machine.

Interestingly, according to IHRSA, the growth in home fitness helps the growth in commercial fitness. More than 65 percent of gym members already own some type of home-fitness equipment. Health club members are three times as likely to own home-fitness equipment as non–health club participants. And fitness-center members who own home-fitness products have higher membership retention rates than those who do not own home equipment. Overall, growth in home fitness supports growth in club fitness and vice versa.

BOTTOM LINE:
THERE'S NO PLACE LIKE HOME!

Bowflex is an excellent strength-training machine specifically designed to be used at home. It's versatile (provides more than sixty different exercises), durable, portable, quiet, requires little maintenance, and is safe. And, using it properly with the correct eating plan, it produces significant results—the same kind of results you get with heavy-duty machines such as Nautilus, MedX, Cybex, and Hammer, which are found in commercial fitness centers.

In many ways, Bowflex at home beats the commercial gym. With Bowflex, there's no drive, no contract to sign, no dress code, no closed doors, no crowds, no feeling stupid, no physique anxiety, no distractions, no wasted time.

Next, Part II describes and illustrates the best Bowflex exercises and organizes them into result-producing routines. After that, Part III covers the science behind building muscle and losing fat. Then, Part IV gets into the specialized programs.

If you're already a Bowflex user and are anxious to embark on one of the specialized programs, here's my suggestion: *Proceed immediately to Part IV and decide on the one that's best for you. Then, go for it!*

Once you've started the program, go back and study Part II for anything you may need brushing up on concerning the Bowflex exercises. Next, thoroughly explore Part III for many helpful hints on getting better results from the muscle-building and fat-loss programs. Finally, Part V shows you how to make more progress, maintain your results, and live leaner and stronger for the rest of your life.

Stay alert and study often on your journey.

PART II EXERCISES

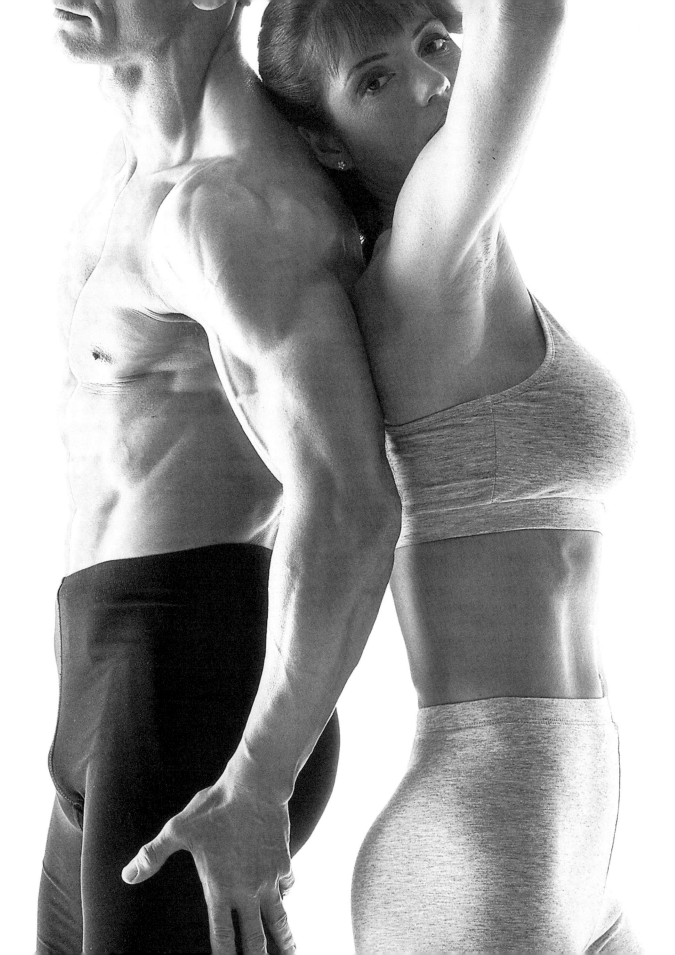

5
STRENGTH-TRAINING BASICS:

REPETITIONS, INTENSITY, & FORM

GREAT TEACHERS . . . WHAT DO they all have in common?

Besides making a subject interesting, they hammer you with the basics.

I was fortunate when growing up to be instructed in reading, writing, arithmetic, and science, as well as chemistry, football, sociology, nutrition, and strength training by ten master teachers. Of those great teachers, two stand out as having an almost daily effect on my life.

The first was a woman named Ilanon Moon, who taught English grammar and composition at my high school in Conroe, Texas. "English," she once declared to me, "is the richest and most varied of all the languages." I was struggling to find the proper synonym to avoid being repetitious in my writing. I was ready to give up and use the same word again. "No," she said. "Ell, you're just being lazy. There's a perfect word just waiting for you. Your job as an educated writer is to find it. Keep thinking."

Moon was right. In five minutes, I had the ideal word.

The second person who influenced me greatly was Arthur Jones, whom I've mentioned several times here. Jones, as the man behind Nautilus exercise equipment, opened doors and pushed me to explore subjects and concepts I would not have delved into without his help.

BACK TO BASICS

Concerning the fundamentals of English grammar and writing, I've heard the voice of Ilanon Moon many times: "The basic rules can be stated on the front and back of one sheet of paper. First and foremost, a student must apply and master those basic rules. But that's not enough. The exceptions to those rules fill more than five hundred pages. Eventually, a writer must study and understand the exceptions. The exceptions add interest, sparkle, and unexpected drama to a page. Effective use of the exceptions separates a good writer from a great writer."

Arthur Jones, in 1974, wrote an article entitled, "All You Need to Know about Strength Training in One Thousand Words." Then, over the next twenty-five years, he published more than a million words about the basics and the exceptions.

To become great, I believe, you need both—the basics and the exceptions. This chapter is about the basics. To get maximum results from strength training on Bowflex, apply the following guidelines:

- Select a resistance on the Power Rods that allows you to perform between 8 and 12 repetitions of each exercise.

- Keep the intensity high by performing each Bowflex exercise until momentary muscular failure.

- Increase the resistance on the Power Rods by 10 pounds when you can perform 12 or more repetitions of any exercise.

- Bend and extend the Power Rod resistance smoothly and slowly during each repetition.

- Work your largest muscles first and smallest muscles last.

- Perform 12 or fewer exercises during each workout.

- Train no more than three times per week.

- Optimize recovery ability, and results, by training less as the body gets stronger.

- Maintain written records—date, exercise, resistance, and repetitions—for each workout.

It's important that you have a complete understanding of each of these basic guidelines.

SELECT A RESISTANCE ON THE POWER RODS THAT ALLOWS YOU TO PERFORM BETWEEN 8 AND 12 REPETITIONS OF EACH EXERCISE

Since the early days of Nautilus, performing between 8 and 12 repetitions has been a mainstay of productive strength training. Occasionally, fewer or more repetitions may be used. But over many years, 8 to 12 has proved to be the best general guideline to follow. The same is true when using a Bowflex machine.

If you perform only 3 or 4 repetitions, your muscles will not be taxed to their limit. On the other hand, if you do 16 to 20 repetitions, you may fail from a lack of oxygen rather than from having reached actual muscular failure. Once again, you would not be taxing your muscles to their limit. The most efficient muscle stimulation occurs when the resistance on the Power Rods allows you to do between 8 and 12 repetitions.

Research shows that optimum strength gains occur when an exercise is at least 40 seconds in duration, but not more than 90 seconds. If you perform 10 repetitions of a given exercise, simple division reveals that each repetition should take from 4 to 9 seconds. An exercise with a short range of movement, such as the Shoulder Shrug or Calf Raise, might require 4 seconds per repetition. An exercise with a long range of movement, such as the Lying Shoulder Pullover or Chest Fly, might take up to 9 seconds or more per repetition. Still, 8 to 12 repetitions is an excellent guideline to use on both short and long range-of-movement exercises.

KEEP THE INTENSITY HIGH BY PERFORMING EACH BOWFLEX EXERCISE UNTIL MOMENTARY MUSCULAR FAILURE

The strength you build—and ultimately the calories you burn—from Bowflex exercise depends on the intensity of your workouts. Research has shown that low-intensity exercise produces little increase in strength and burns few calories during and after the workout. Strength improvement and fat burning is best produced by high-intensity exercise.

"High intensity" means extreme effort. Maximum intensity occurs when a muscle is pulling as hard as it possibly can. Ideally, this should happen during the 8th, 9th, 10th, 11th, 12th, or at most 13th repetition, if the resistance has been appropriately set. By the last repetition, the muscles involved should barely be able to complete the range. When movement stops, despite your best efforts, then you have reached what is called "momentary muscular failure," which is your goal.

This maximum effort sends your body a signal that says, in effect, *Grow larger and stronger before this happens again*. Intense exercise stimulates compensatory buildup in the form of added muscle tissue, which aids the body in coping more successfully with similar stress in the future.

Performing a Bowflex exercise to the point that you cannot possibly do one more repetition—the point of momentary muscular failure—is high intensity. When you feel you can't do another, try again. Try until no forward progress is possible.

When a Bowflex exercise is performed in a high-intensity manner, one set—and only one set—gives your involved muscle group optimum stimulation. It is usually not necessary to do multiple sets.

POWER ROD RESISTANCE INCREASES BY 10 POUNDS WHEN YOU CAN PERFORM 12 OR MORE REPETITIONS

Progression is the central idea behind strength training. Continuing to do what you can already do won't make you stronger. During each follow-up workout, you must attempt to do more repetitions until you reach 12, then you will have to add more resistance.

The lightest Power Rod on a Bowflex machine is 5 pounds. Since most exercises are performed bilaterally, Power Rods on both sides of the machine are required. Thus, the lightest progression that you can make on these exercises is 10 pounds.

For example, on the bench press exercise, let's say you can do 10 repetitions with 40 pounds of Power Rods on each side. That's a total of 80 pounds, which is recorded on your workout card as 80/10. On the following workout, you do 12 repetitions and almost 13, with the same 80 pounds. That's written down as 80/12. Several days later, during your next workout, add a 5-pound Power Rod to each side before you attempt the bench press. If you're like most people, you'll probably complete 7 or 8 repetitions with the new resistance, which is now 90 pounds.

Very simply, your goal for each exercise on every workout is to make small progressions—in the number of repetitions, the amount of resistance, or both.

BEND AND EXTEND THE POWER ROD RESISTANCE SMOOTHLY AND SLOWLY DURING EACH REPETITION

Inertia is the tendency of a weight or mass, if in motion, to keep moving in the same direction. The quantity of this motion is called momentum. Momentum is a big problem with free weights and weight-stack machines because of the inclination most trainees have to lift the weight too quickly. Because there is no weight stack involved in a Bowflex machine, there is very little momentum in a repetition. But there is potential momentum in a moving arm, leg, or other body part connected to a Bowflex handle—if the movement is performed too

HOW TO BREATHE WHILE STRENGTH TRAINING

During a Bowflex exercise, the idea is to concentrate on the muscles involved, not on your breathing. If you simply forget about *how* to breathe but remember to *keep doing* it, your breathing will take care of itself and supply your body with adequate oxygen—especially if your heart rate is high enough. There are, however, points along the range of motion of every Bowflex exercise where it's easier to breathe in or out. Your subconscious mind will identify these points and coordinate your breathing quite efficiently and naturally.

It's essential, however, to refrain from holding your breath during the most intense repetitions. Keeping your air passages closed while straining can cause something called the Valsalva effect, which may cause a blackout or headache. Do not hold your breath. Open your mouth if necessary and *keep breathing*.

fast. That's why smooth, slow repetitions are preferred.

When you pull or push on the handles of a Bowflex machine, the Power Rods bend and the muscles involved contract concentrically, or positively. When the Power Rods extend, the same muscles relax eccentrically, or negatively. This is similar to lifting a barbell or dumbbell, or using a weight-stack machine. Lifting the weight is positive; lowering the weight is negative. An exercise on a Bowflex machine may differ from a free weight exercise because the direction of movement is not necessarily more effective when you're moving straight up. With a barbell, for example, straight up is harder. With a Bowflex exercise, the direction of movement may be up, down, horizontal, or anywhere in between. The Power Rods do not need an assist from gravity to operate. Regardless of the direction, you still get effective resistance.

It is necessary to understand this to correctly perform a repetition on a Bowflex machine.

During the early Nautilus days, 1973–1980, I instructed trainees to take approximately 6 seconds to do a repetition on a Nautilus machine—2 seconds on the positive and 4 seconds on the negative (2/4). Taking twice as long in the negative worked pretty well on machines that had carried a lot of mechanical friction. The early Nautilus machines contained bushings in the pivot points, as opposed to today's almost frictionless bearings. On today's Nautilus machines, I recommend both the positive and negative phases be performed at the same approximate speed. Depending on the range of movement of the exercise, that speed can be from 4 seconds (2/2) on a wrist curl to 14 seconds (7/7) on a pullover machine. An average of all the machines creates a guideline of 4 seconds on the positive and 4 seconds on the negative (4/4).

The Bowflex exercises vary in a similar way to the Nautilus machines, with one primary exception. Because of less momentum on a Bowflex machine, a repetition can be a shade faster. That's why the overall guideline of 3 seconds positive and 3 seconds negative is recommended (3/3). Generally, the idea is to keep the movement smooth and slow, especially at the turnarounds, where the movement changes direction from positive to negative and from negative to positive.

Never try to jerk, bounce, yank, throw, or kick into the handles, bars, or pads of any Bowflex exercise. Doing so is unproductive, dangerous, and may lead to an injury.

During any strength-training exercise, always practice the following: *Move slowly, change direction smoothly, and start and stop gradually.* Your results will be faster, greater, and safer.

WORK YOUR LARGEST MUSCLES FIRST AND YOUR SMALLEST MUSCLES LAST

As an assignment, let's examine the following three sequences for working body parts and decide which one will produce the best strength-training results.

• Popularity Listing: biceps, triceps, chest, waist, shoulders, back, and legs. Do three days per week.

• Largest to Smallest: legs, back, chest, shoulders, triceps, biceps, and waist. Do three days per week.

• Lower-Body and Upper-Body Split: Lower—thighs, calves, and waist; Upper—chest, back, shoulders, biceps, and triceps. Do three days per week on lower body and three days per week on upper body, or six days per week in total. Now for the analysis.

Popularity listing. This is the way most men train. The emphasis is on the show muscles: biceps, triceps, and chest. Recently, the waist has received a lot of attention, so many men often work their waist first. Either way, there are several problems behind such ordering.

First, the arms and chest contain much smaller muscles than those of the thighs and hips. Working the smaller muscles first usually leads to a less than all-out effort when you finally get to exercising the larger muscles. I've found that it's to your advantage to train your largest, strongest muscles first, that is, when you are the freshest and most motivated. You'll get a better spillover, or indirect effect, by proceeding from the largest to the smallest muscles than you will by proceeding from the smallest to the largest muscles.

Second, your largest, strongest muscles—the gluteals, quadriceps, and hamstrings—form the foundation or core of building a great upper body. Evidently, your body allows only a certain degree of disproportionate development. In other words, you can never reach your genetic potential in your upper body by working only your upper body. A certain amount of lower-body exercise is required. In fact, frequently concentrating on your lower body is one of the secrets to massive upper-body development. Thus, I usually recommend that you exercise your lower body before your upper body.

Largest to smallest. This is the best way to sequence your workout. It probably doesn't make too much difference about the torso ordering: chest before back, back before shoulders, shoulders before chest? They are all approximately the same size. I do, however, like to separate two pulling movements with a pushing exercise, or two pushing exercises with a pulling movement.

Lower-body and upper-body split. There are dozens of ways to divide the body into various routines and doing so seems to be the most popular way for advanced bodybuilders to train. Most of these split routines require spending at least twice as much time training compared to working the entire body each session. Split routines soon lead to overtraining and inefficient results.

Years of experience have taught me that the human body operates best as a whole, not as separate parts. Even when you try only to work your lower body, you still involve your upper body to a moderate degree. You certainly can't organize other systems within your body to eat, digest, eliminate, and sleep for this half or that half. Train your body as a unit, rest it as a unit—for maximum results.

PERFORM 12 OR FEWER EXERCISES DURING EACH WORKOUT

If each Bowflex exercise is done properly in a high-intensity fashion, brief workouts must be the rule. Twelve is the maximum number of exercises that you should perform. Divide them into two to six for the lower body and four to eight for the upper body.

A set of 12 repetitions should take no more than 90 seconds to perform. Allowing one minute between exercises, you should be able to perform twelve Bowflex exercises in fewer than 30 minutes. As you work yourself into better condition, the time between exercises should be reduced. It's possible, with the help of an assistant, to go through an entire workout of twelve Bowflex exercises in fewer than 20 minutes. Such a workout develops not only muscular strength and joint flexibility but also a high level of cardiovascular endurance.

TRAIN NO MORE THAN THREE TIMES PER WEEK

There should be at least two days, or approximately forty-eight hours, but not more than four days, or approximately ninety-six hours, between Bowflex workouts. Remember, exercise is the stimulation. Your body must be permitted to overcompensate and become stronger.

An every-other-day, three-times-per-week Bowflex program also provides your body with the needed irregularity of training. A first workout is performed on Monday, a second on Wednesday, and a third on

Friday. On Sunday, your body expects and prepares for a fourth workout, but it does not come. Instead, it comes a day later, Monday, when your body is not expecting it. This schedule prevents your body from falling into a regular routine. Growth is stimulated because your system is never able to adjust to the irregularity of training.

OPTIMIZE RECOVERY ABILITY AND RESULTS BY TRAINING LESS AS YOUR BODY GETS STRONGER

Recovery ability is the wide array of chemical reactions that must occur inside your body for your system to compensate, not only from a hard workout but to overcompensate and become stronger. *Important:* Your recovery ability does not increase in proportion to your body's ability to get stronger. Arthur Jones used to graph recovery ability as 50 units and strength potential as 300 units. His graph revealed a 1:6 recovery/strength ratio for most people. To reach your strength potential requires rest and recovery time. As you get stronger, you must concentrate on doing less.

Less overall exercise is accomplished in two ways: *by reducing the number of workouts per week* and *by doing fewer exercises per workout.*

THE BEST OF MORE THAN SEVENTY-EIGHT BOWFLEX EXERCISES

If you count all the variations, and include the attachments, more than seventy-eight exercises may be performed on the Bowflex Ultimate machine. With the Bowflex Power Pro, sixty exercises are possible. If you've purchased any Bowflex machine, you can refer to the *Owner's Manual and Fitness Guide* for descriptions and illustrations of all the possible exercises. Or, you can log on to the Web site, www.Bowflex.com, and view or download any of the illustrated manuals.

In the next three chapters, I focus on what I consider to be the best Bowflex exercises. Since a Bowflex machine has to adapt to so many exercises, some are better performed in certain positions than in others. Also, some exercises require a long range of movement and thus a complete bend of the Power Rods; others do not. *Best*, when used in the context of Bowflex exercises, *means that the selected movement has good stabilization, and usually, a long range of movement*. And in this book, *best* means it's one of the Bowflex exercises that I recommend in the ensuing chapters.

There are twenty-three best exercises in all, and they are subdivided into five for the lower body (chapter 6), ten for the back, chest, and shoulders (chapter 7), and eight for the arms and abdominals (chapter 8). For consistency, the Bowflex Ultimate machine is used to illustrate all of the recommended exercises.

Let's say your progress has come to a halt. You've been training several months, three times per week, and you've been performing one set of twelve different Bowflex exercises. You're on a plateau, however. Your repetitions will not increase. Here are my suggestions.

First. Reduce your training frequency. Drop from three to two and a half days per week. To accomplish this, look at a two-week segment. It becomes easy to manage if you go from six times in two weeks to five times in two weeks. Instead of Monday, Wednesday, Friday, Monday, Wednesday, Friday, the schedule becomes Monday, Thursday, Sunday, Wednesday, Saturday. Then, the following two-week segment moves to Tuesday, Friday, Monday, Thursday, Sunday. Simply get out a blank calendar, allow seventy-two hours between workouts, and mark your training days.

Second. You're now performing your twelve-exercise routine five times in two weeks. As you get stronger, another plateau stands in your pathway. This is the time to do fewer exercises. Instead of twelve, try ten—and continue doing ten until you reach a plateau again.

Third. This plateau is a signal that you should reduce your frequency. Go from five times in two weeks to four times in two weeks, or twice a week.

Fourth. Another plateau calls for fewer exercises. Try eight instead of ten.

Fifth. I've never trained an athlete or advanced bodybuilder—and I've trained some big, strong men—who needed to reduce past the level of three times in two weeks or fewer than five exercises per routine. I suppose there are a few Goliaths somewhere who might thrive on such a schedule. I'd like to hear from you if you think you're in that category, or if you know anyone who is.

MAINTAIN WRITTEN RECORDS FOR EACH WORKOUT

You'd be surprised by the number of people who strength-train and don't keep records of what they do. Sure, they follow some type of plan, but they don't write it down or record their resistance and repetitions on any exercise. Don't let yourself fall into this group.

Only by keeping accurate records can you determine your progress. Each Bowflex workout should be recorded on a card, which may resemble the one on page 53. For a blank workout card, which you can photocopy, turn to page 285.

The first entry for the Leg Curl is 70/10. This means the trainee performed 10 repetitions with 70 pounds of Power Rods. Thirteen repetitions were done during the third workout, so the resistance was increased by 10 pounds for the fourth workout. The upward-pointing arrow is a reminder to increase the resistance at the next workout. Any of the other exercises listed on the card can be documented in a similar manner and examined in detail.

Reviewing your workout card periodically will allow you to assess your week-by-week progress. After all, that's precisely what you are trying to do: make progress and get stronger.

Remember, it's important to maintain written records of all your Bowflex workouts.

PRE-PERFORMANCE PREPARATION

Before getting into each exercise, there are a few things that you need to know and do.

Study your Bowflex machine. It's important that you get to know your Bowflex machine. Please locate your *Owner's Manual and Fitness Guide* and review pages 1–7. Or you may log on to the Web site www.Bowflex.com and read or download the manual to your computer. You'll find detailed information about each machine that Bowflex manufactures, with all the salient parts noted. Study carefully how the Power Rods are organized and how they hook and unhook from the cables. Try the wide and narrow

pulley system, if it is a part of your machine. Make sure you understand the workout bench and how to adjust it for the different exercises. Also, become familiar with the hand grips, straps, and belts—and how they work. There's also a page devoted to folding and moving your Bowflex machine, as well as maintenance of it. Review that, too.

Practice correct posture during each exercise. Correct posture on most Bowflex exercises means keeping your chest up, abdominals tight, and maintaining a slight arch in your lower back. Your head should be in a neutral (not strained) position on most exercises. When seated, always keep both feet flat on the platform or floor. When standing, your feet need to be at least a shoulder width apart for stability. Also, when standing keep a soft bend in your knees during each exercise.

Review safety precautions. In your *Owner's Manual* there is a page devoted to safety instructions. Please review this page and pay particular attention to the following: Keep out of the path of the Power Rods when exercising, caution observers to stand clear of the Power Rods, do not stand directly over the top of Power Rods when hooking and unhooking them, tighten the adjustable pulley system's pins before use, and make sure the spring-lock seat pin is securely fastened and the bench is firmly in place before use.

WARMING UP AND COOLING DOWN

Evidence supports the need for a general warm-up as a safeguard against injury. Almost any sequence of light calisthenic movements—such as head rotation, side bend, trunk twist, and walking in place—can precede a Bowflex workout. Or, best of all, you can warm up on your Bowflex machine by performing a simple movement called Aerobic Rowing. Three minutes of Aerobic Rowing should be sufficient for a general warming up. Specific warming up of each body part is built into each Bowflex exercise during the first 3 or 4 repetitions.

A cooldown period after your workout is also important. This prevents blood from pooling in your exercised muscles. Once again, Aerobic Rowing is the movement of choice. Or, after your last Bowflex exercise, you may choose to cool down by walking around the workout area, getting a drink of water, and moving your arms in slow circles. Another 3 minutes or so in either mode gradually shifts your mind and body into a more relaxed state.

Here's how to do the Aerobic Rowing, which requires only a light resistance on the Power Rods:

• Remove the bench and set aside.

• Unlock the rowing seat and place in free-sliding mode.

• Sit on the seat facing the Power Rods.

• Grasp the handles and keep your arms straight to front.

• Position the arches of your feet on the footrest of the machine with your knees bent.

• Sit tall.

• Straighten your knees while bending your arms in a rowing fashion as the seat moves backward.

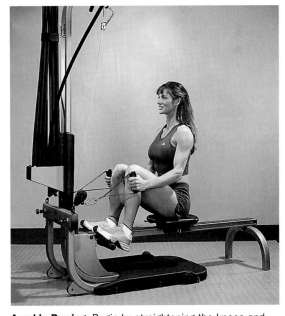

Aerobic Rowing: Begin by straightening the knees and bending the arms simultaneously, then bending the knees and straightening the arms.

• Do not straighten your knees completely.

• Return to the bent-knee position while keeping your torso erect.

• Repeat in a smooth, controlled manner as a warm-up or cooldown for approximately 3 minutes.

LOOKING AHEAD

Review this chapter often during your initial Bowflex training sessions. Doing so will arm you with sufficient basic information, which, when it is combined with the instructional details in chapters 6, 7, and 8, will head you down the road to optimum results.

Not only do you need to master the basics, as both Ilanon Moon and Arthur Jones have taught me, but eventually you must have a grasp of the exceptions. It requires another 230 pages to cover the exceptions.

The best is yet to come.

EXERCISE	Date	3/3	3/5	3/7	3/10		
	Body weight	171.5	170	169.5	168.5		
1. Leg Curl		70/10	70/11	70/13↑	80/8		
2. Leg Extension		80/9	80/10	80/11	80/12↑		
3. Bench Press		80/7	80/9	80/10	80/11		
4. Seated Row		90/10	90/12↑	100/9	100/8		
5. Lying Shoulder Pullover		60/11	60/13↑	70/10	70/11		
6. Seated Abdominal Crunch		60/10	60/11	60/12↑	70/8		
7.							
8.							
9.							
10.							
11.							
12.							

Dr. Ellington Darden's BOWFLEX BODY PLAN

6

LOWER-BODY EXERCISES:

FOR PERFORMANCE & APPEARANCE

THE MUSCLES OF THE HIPS, THIGHS, and calves compose what is generally called the lower body. The lower body houses your largest and strongest muscles and there are many reasons to keep them in good working condition. Strong lower-body muscles:

• Protect your hip, knee, and ankle joints from a lifetime of walking, running, climbing, bending, lifting, and jumping

• Help to prevent injury in many sports that involve the legs

• Allow you to perform better in almost every sport, from acrobatics and badminton to softball and yachting

• Permit you to work your cardiovascular system efficiently

• Are more and more important—as you age—for balance, getting up from a chair, and general mobility

• Burn more calories under both working and resting conditions

• Have better shape, contour, and visual appeal, especially in shorts, than do weak lower-body muscles

There is really no good reason not to work your lower body.

HIP, THIGH, AND CALF EXERCISES

Great, you're now ready for a look at the best Bowflex exercises for your lower body:

Leg Curl

Leg Extension

Leg Press

Seated Leg Curl

Seated (Straight Leg) Calf Raise

For each exercise I will describe the Targeted Body Part, Joint Motion, Muscles Worked, Pulley Position, Starting Position, Action, and Training Tips.

LEG CURL

TARGETED BODY PART: BACK THIGHS

JOINT MOTION: KNEE FLEXION

MUSCLES WORKED: HAMSTRINGS

PULLEY POSITION: LEG-EXTENSION/LEG-CURL ATTACHMENT

STARTING POSITION

- Attach bench to seat of leg unit. Rest other end on rail, so that it forms a slight decline.
- Lie facedown on bench with back ankles under upper roller pads.
- Make sure knees are near pivot point of movement arm.
- Place hands on side of rail or bench for stability.

ACTION

- Curl heels by bending knees and try to touch roller pads to buttocks.
- Pause in the contracted position.
- Lower slowly and return to the starting position.
- Repeat for required repetitions.

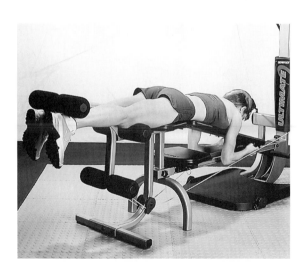 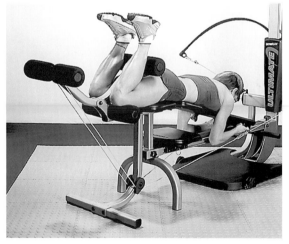

TRAINING TIPS

- Keep calf and foot muscles relaxed during movement. Do not extend toes. • Maintain a neutral position of head and neck during exercise.

LEG EXTENSION

TARGETED BODY PART: FRONT THIGHS

JOINT MOTION: KNEE EXTENSION

MUSCLES WORKED: QUADRICEPS

PULLEY POSITION: LEG-EXTENSION/LEG-CURL ATTACHMENT

STARTING POSITION

- Sit on high seat facing away from Power Rods with knees near pivot point.
- Wedge feet and shins under roller pads.
- Position thighs at hip width with kneecaps straight to front.
- Place hands on sides of seat bottom.

ACTION

- Straighten legs smoothly by moving feet forward and upward until knees are fully extended.
- Pause in contracted position.
- Return slowly to starting position.
- Repeat for required repetitions.

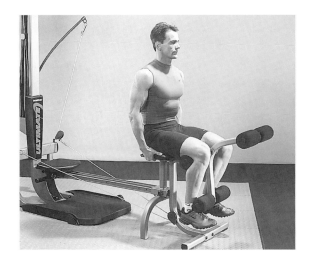 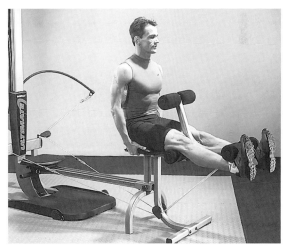

TRAINING TIPS

- Lift and lower roller pads under control. Do not kick into pads. Always adhere to good form. • Keep feet relaxed during movement. • Try to relax neck and face on latter repetitions.

LEG PRESS

TARGETED BODY PART: BUTTOCKS, BACK THIGHS, AND FRONT THIGHS

JOINT MOTIONS: HIP EXTENSION AND KNEE EXTENSION

MUSCLES WORKED: GLUTEALS, HAMSTRINGS, AND QUADRICEPS

PULLEY POSITION: NARROW

STARTING POSITION

- Remove bench and set aside.
- Unlock rowing seat and place in free-sliding mode.
- Sit on seat facing Power Rods.
- Attach leg press belt and adjust properly around hips.
- Place feet on upright pulley frame or footrests.
- Straighten legs, but do not lock knees
- Rest hands on sides of belt.

ACTION

- Bend hips and knees and slide toward Power Rods slowly.
- Make the turnaround gradually.
- Press smoothly into position with knees almost straight.
- Repeat for required repetitions.

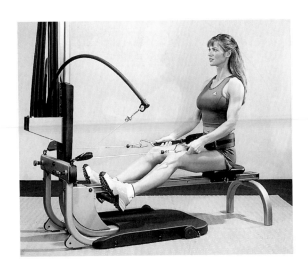 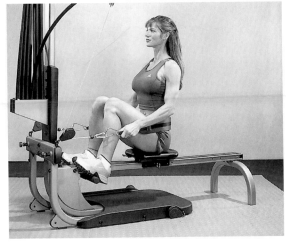

TRAINING TIPS

- Keep knees pointed in same direction as feet. • Focus on pressing through calf bones into frame of machine, rather than simply moving seat backward. • Stop short of locking knees. • Move slowly during all repetitions. Do not fire out or use momentum.

SEATED LEG CURL

TARGETED BODY PART: BACK THIGHS

JOINT MOTIONS: KNEE FLEXION WITH HIP FLEXION

MUSCLES WORKED: HAMSTRINGS

PULLEY POSITION: NARROW

STARTING POSITION

- Remove bench and set aside.
- Unlock rowing seat and place in free-sliding mode.
- Attach one end of belt to pulley.
- Sit on seat facing away from Power Rods.
- Draw belt across midsection and attach free end to other pulley.
- Slide forward and secure heels at end of machine.
- Place hands on edge of seat.

ACTION

- Pull with heels on end of machine.
- Slide seat forward smoothly as knees bend.
- Pause in the contracted position.
- Allow legs to straighten slowly.
- Repeat bending and straightening for required repetitions.

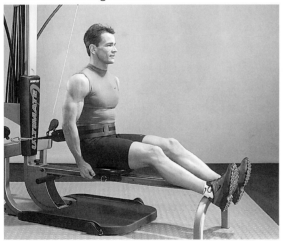
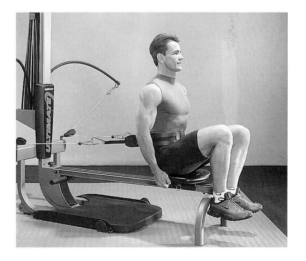

TRAINING TIPS

- Keep ankles in flexed position throughout movement. • Do not bounce in and out of contracted or stretched position. Stay in control of each repetition.

SEATED (STRAIGHT LEG) CALF RAISE

TARGETED BODY PART: BACK CALF

JOINT MOTION: ANKLE EXTENSION

MUSCLES WORKED: GASTROCNEMIUS AND SOLEUS

PULLEY POSITION: NARROW

STARTING POSITION

- Remove bench and set aside.
- Unlock rowing seat and place in free-sliding mode.
- Sit on seat facing Power Rods.
- Adjust leg press belt around hips.
- Put balls of feet on upright pulley frame.
- Straighten legs, but do not lock knees.
- Place hands on sides of belt.

ACTION

- Press balls of feet into frame and smoothly move heels toward knees. Doing so slides the seat backward.
- Pause in contracted position.
- Return to starting position for a slow stretch.
- Repeat for required repetitions.

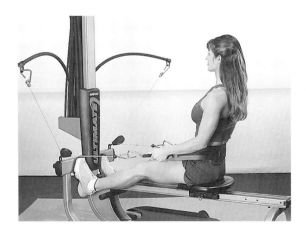 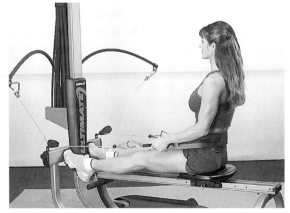

TRAINING TIPS

- Do not change hip or knee position. Focus on moving ankles. • Try to extend on big toes in contracted position for more calf involvement.

7

BACK, CHEST, & SHOULDER EXERCISES:

WHAT'S BEST FOR THE TORSO

THE LARGEST MUSCLES OF YOUR BACK, chest, and shoulders, in order, are the latissimus dorsi, pectoralis major, and deltoids. Each of these muscles crosses your shoulder joint and attaches to the upper-arm bone. As a result, these muscles allow a variety of arm movements.

Pulling exercises with the arms involve the latissimus dorsi muscles. When developed, these sweeping muscles provide a pleasing V shape to the upper torso, especially when viewed from the back.

The pectoralis majors fan across the front of the chest. These muscles aid pushing movements of the arms. Strong pectoral muscles add torso thickness from both the front and the side.

Well-developed deltoids contribute impressive roundness to the tops of your shoulders. Lifting your arms sideways and pressing overhead involve the deltoids.

Strong, well-developed latissimus dorsi, pectoralis major, and deltoid muscles not only look good, they provide structural integrity to the shoulder joints. Next to the knees, the shoulder joints are the most vulnerable to the effects of aging. You can do a lot to prevent the effects of aging by keeping your major torso muscles active and strong.

A Bowflex machine offers more than thirty different exercises for the back, chest, and shoulders. For a full discussion of all of these movements, you'll want to refer to your *Owner's Manual and Fitness Guide*, or log on to the Web site www.Bowflex.com.

The best exercises for the back, chest, and shoulders are as follows:

BACK

Seated Row

Lying Lat Pulldown

Reverse Grip Pulldown

CHEST

Bench Press

Chest Fly

Incline Bench Press

Lying Shoulder Pullover

SHOULDERS

Standing Lateral Raise

Seated Shoulder Press

Shoulder Shrug

Let's take a close look at each exercise.

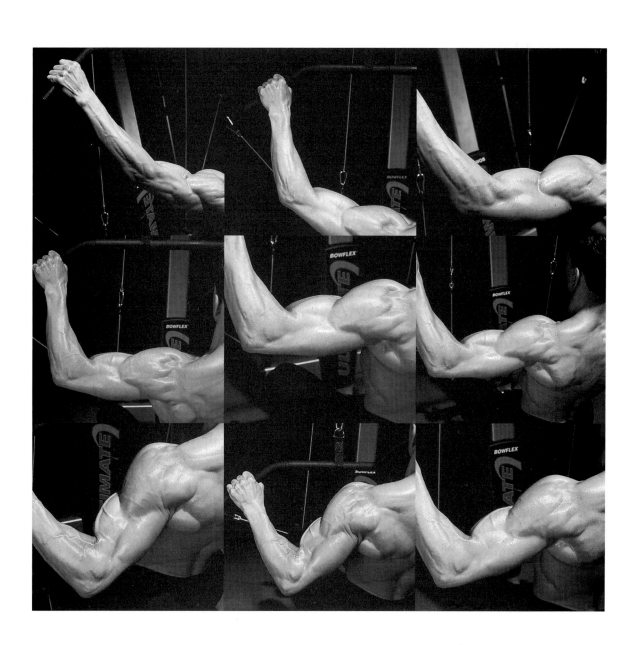

SEATED ROW

TARGETED BODY PART: UPPER BACK

JOINT MOTIONS: SHOULDER EXTENSION AND ELBOW FLEXION

MUSCLES WORKED: LATISSIMUS DORSI AND BICEPS

PULLEY POSITION: NARROW

STARTING POSITION

- Straddle bench and sit facing the Power Rods.
- Grasp handles with palms facing each other.
- Place feet on platform and bend knees.
- Sit tall and tighten abdominals. Do not slouch during movement.

ACTION

- Begin by pinching shoulder blades together and at the same time pulling arms back and inward toward sides of torso.
- Move upper arms past torso and pause in contracted position.
- Return slowly to starting position by straightening arms.
- Repeat for required repetitions.

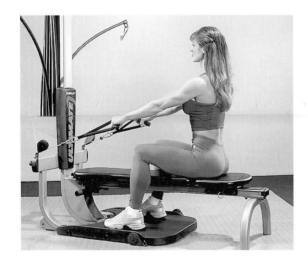 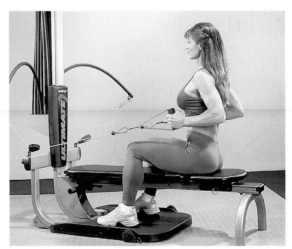

TRAINING TIPS

- Keep chest lifted during all repetitions. • Do not lean forward by rounding shoulders. Sit erect.

LYING LAT PULLDOWN

TARGETED BODY PART: LATISSIMUS DORSI

JOINT MOTION: SHOULDER ADDUCTION

MUSCLES WORKED: LATISSIMUS DORSI WITHOUT BICEPS INVOLVEMENT

PULLEY POSITION: WIDE

STARTING POSITION

- Sit on bench facing away from Power Rods.
- Lie on back, grasp a handle, slip arm through handle, and tighten cuff just past elbow. Do the same with other arm.
- Slide body away from Power Rods until arms are extended. Bend knees and place feet flat on floor.
- Keep arms wide and out to sides.

ACTION

- Pull upper arms sideward toward waist.
- Pause in contracted position.
- Return to starting position.
- Repeat for required repetitions.

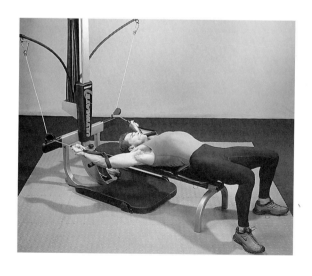 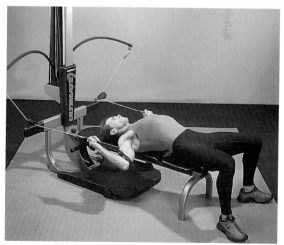

TRAINING TIPS

- Make sure cuff is tight around upper arms. • Move upper arms in a sideward or horizontal arc, not forward and down.

REVERSE GRIP PULLDOWN

TARGETED BODY PART: UPPER BACK

JOINT MOTIONS: SHOULDER EXTENSION AND ELBOW FLEXION

MUSCLES WORKED: LATISSIMUS DORSI AND BICEPS

PULLEY POSITION: NARROW

STARTING POSITION

- Straddle bench facing Power Rods.
- Grasp bar with palms up and hands shoulder width apart and sit down.
- Position knees under pulleys with feet flat on platform and arms extended overhead.

ACTION

- Pull lat bar smoothly to chest.
- Pause in contracted position.
- Return slowly to starting position.
- Repeat for required repetitions.

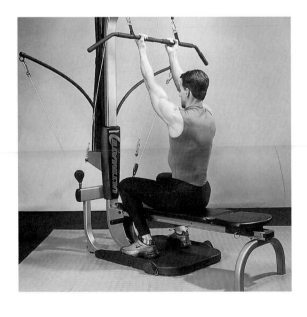 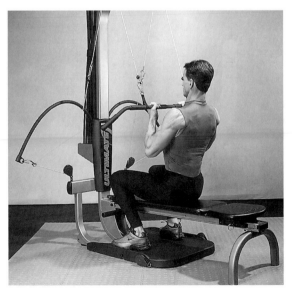

TRAINING TIPS

- Stay erect during all repetitions. Maintain feet flat on floor. • Do not lean back with torso in contracted position. Keep chest up.

BENCH PRESS

TARGETED BODY PART: FRONT CHEST

JOINT MOTIONS: SHOULDER HORIZONTAL ADDUCTION AND ELBOW EXTENSION

MUSCLES WORKED: PECTORALIS MAJOR, ANTERIOR DELTOID, AND TRICEPS

PULLEY POSITION: WIDE

STARTING POSITION

- Adjust bench to 45-degree position and sit facing away from Power Rods.
- Grasp handles and bend elbows until hands are near chest.
- Position feet flat on floor.
- Straighten arms to front with handles shoulder width apart.
- Keep shoulder blades pinched together throughout movement.

ACTION

- Bend elbows outward while slowly lowering handles until thumbs are near shoulders.
- Return smoothly to starting position with arms straight in front and shoulder width apart.
- Repeat for required repetitions.

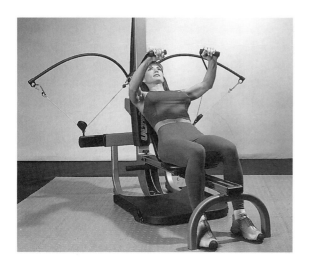
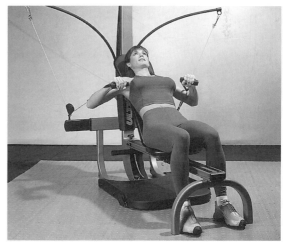

TRAINING TIPS

- Be careful of range of motion in stretched position. Don't be excessive. Stop when elbows are slightly behind shoulders. • Improve chest involvement by keeping shoulder blades pinched together through entire movement.

CHEST FLY

TARGETED BODY PART: FRONT CHEST

JOINT MOTION: SHOULDER HORIZONTAL ADDUCTION WITH ELBOW STABILIZED

MUSCLES WORKED: PECTORALIS MAJOR

PULLEY POSITION: WIDE

STARTING POSITION

- Adjust bench to 45-degree position and sit facing away from Power Rods.
- Grasp handles and bend arms until hands are near chest.
- Position feet flat on floor.
- Straighten arms to front and bring handles together with palms facing each other.
- Pinch shoulder blades together throughout movement.

ACTION

- Move handles outward while keeping elbows slightly bent.
- Continue lowering handles until elbows are slightly below shoulders.
- Try to pull handles back to over-chest position with pectorals, rather than push with triceps.
- Repeat for required repetitions.

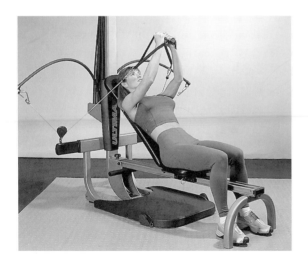 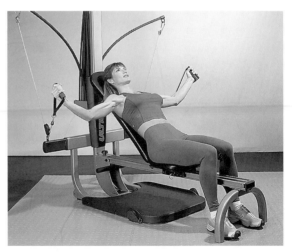

TRAINING TIPS

- Begin with moderate resistance and practice good form. • Do not stretch excessively in the bottom position. • Keep elbows slightly bent and stable during entire movement.

INCLINE BENCH PRESS

TARGETED BODY PART: UPPER CHEST

JOINT MOTIONS: SHOULDER HORIZONTAL ADDUCTION AND ELBOW EXTENSION

MUSCLES WORKED: PECTORALIS MAJOR, ANTERIOR DELTOID, AND TRICEPS

PULLEY POSITION: WIDE

STARTING POSITION

- Adjust bench to 45-degree position and sit facing away from Power Rods.
- Grasp handles and bend arms until hands are near chest.
- Position feet flat on floor.
- Straighten arms to front with handles shoulder width apart.
- Raise arms another 10 to 15 degrees above normal bench press.
- Keep shoulder blades pinched together throughout movement.

ACTION

- Move elbows outward while bending elbows and slowly lower handles until thumbs are near shoulders.
- Return smoothly to starting position with arms straight and handles shoulder width apart.
- Repeat for required repetitions.

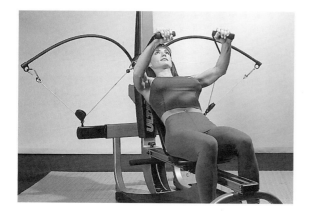 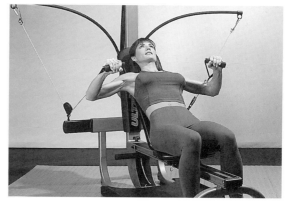

TRAINING TIPS

- Control range of motion, especially in bottom position. Make sure hands travel only slightly behind shoulders.
- Maintain slight arch in lower back throughout movement.

LYING SHOULDER PULLOVER

TARGETED BODY PART: UPPER BACK AND CHEST

JOINT MOTION: SHOULDER EXTENSION WITH ELBOW STABILIZED

MUSCLES WORKED: LATISSIMUS DORSI AND PECTORALIS MAJOR

PULLEY POSITION: NARROW

STARTING POSITION

- Lie on back with head toward Power Rods.
- Scoot down bench until arms can extend overhead without hitting frame.
- Keep knees bent and feet flat on floor.
- Grasp handles with palms facing ceiling.

ACTION

- Move handles in arcs upward and then downward.
- Do not bend elbows. Keep them straight.
- Continue until handles are by hips.
- Return slowly to starting position by reversing the arcs.
- Repeat for required repetitions.

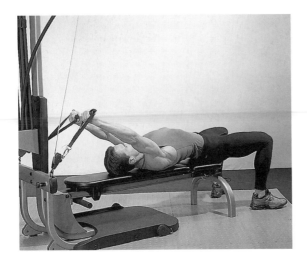 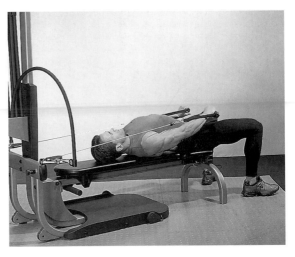

TRAINING TIPS

- Arch midback during pulling, but not excessively. • Anchor feet under machine, if necessary.

STANDING LATERAL RAISE

TARGETED BODY PART: SIDE SHOULDERS

JOINT MOTION: SHOULDER ABDUCTION WITH ELBOW STABILIZED

MUSCLE WORKED: MIDDLE DELTOID

PULLEY POSITION: NARROW

STARTING POSITION

- Remove bench and set aside.
- Straddle rail and face Power Rods.
- Grasp a handle and spread cuff. Slide hand through so pad rests on back of hand. Tighten. Repeat.
- Stand with arms hanging almost in line with cables.
- Stabilize wrists with palms facing each other.
- Lean forward approximately 20 degrees.

ACTION

- Raise handles and arms sideways, while keeping a slight bend in elbows.
- Continue until handles are level with shoulders and pause.
- Lower slowly to the starting position.
- Repeat for required repetitions.

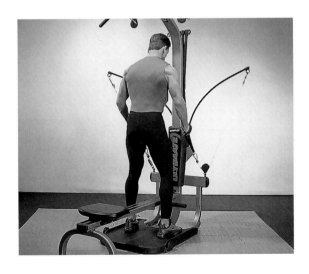 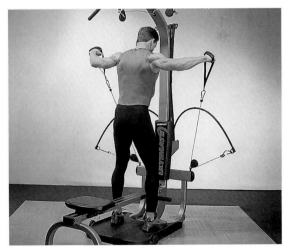

TRAINING TIPS

• Do not shrug shoulders at start. • Maintain leaning-forward position during both lifting and lowering. • Do not rotate arms or hands during movement. Keep palms facing down with elbows slightly bent.

SEATED SHOULDER PRESS

TARGETED BODY PART: SHOULDERS

JOINT MOTIONS: SHOULDER ABDUCTION AND ELBOW EXTENSION

MUSCLES WORKED: DELTOIDS AND TRICEPS

PULLEY POSITION: WIDE

STARTING POSITION

- Sit on bench facing away from Power Rods.
- Scoot back against frame for hip-torso support.
- Grasp handles and bring to shoulders with palms facing away from machine.
- Bend knees and place feet flat on platform.
- Maintain slight arch in lower back.

ACTION

- Press handles smoothly overhead.
- Return slowly to starting position with handles just above shoulder level.
- Repeat for required repetitions.

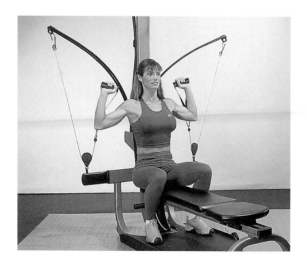 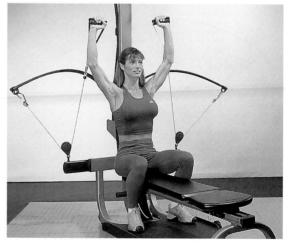

TRAINING TIPS

- Do not increase arch in lower back during movement. Maintain tight abdominals. • Keep handles shoulder-width apart.
- Relax face and neck during last repetitions.

SHOULDER SHRUG

TARGETED BODY PART: UPPER BACK AND NECK

JOINT MOTION: SCAPULAR ELEVATION

MUSCLE WORKED: TRAPEZIUS

PULLEY POSITION: NARROW

STARTING POSITION

- Remove bench and set aside.
- Straddle rail and face Power Rods.
- Grasp handles and stand with palms facing each other.
- Keep elbows straight and do not bend them during movement.

ACTION

- Shrug shoulders smoothly and try to touch shoulders to ears.
- Pause in contracted position.
- Return slowly to starting position.
- Repeat for required repetitions.

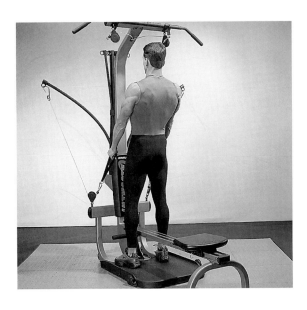 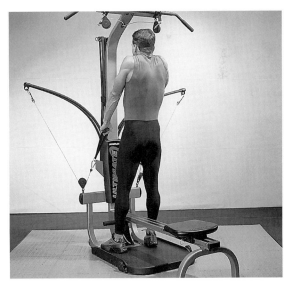

TRAINING TIPS

• Do not lean forward or backward during movement. Do not move head or neck. Stand tall. • Do not grip handles excessively. Do not bend elbows. Use hands and arms as hooks.

8
ARM & ABDOMINAL EXERCISES:
FOR STRENGTH & MUSCULARITY

IN ALMOST EVERY GYM, fitness magazine, and Internet discussion board related to exercise, *arms* and *abdominals* are the most popular topics. But why?

Perhaps the biggest reason that arms are so popular is that they are highly visible. All other body parts can be hidden with clothes, but the arms are often uncovered. Especially for men, large, muscular arms are associated with athletic success. Many fitness-minded women also train their arms for size and shape. Arms that look like weak sticks or hanging blobs are certainly not in style for either sex.

In some circles, attractive abdominals are even more popular than muscular arms. It used to be that being thin was enough. In the 1980s, that started to change. Women's bodybuilding began to catch on when champions Rachel McLish and Cory Everson displayed their lean, chiseled midsections. And then Sylvester Stallone transformed his bulky physique in *Rocky*, in what seemed like only a few months, into rippling *Rambo* abs.

The race was on after that. In the mid-1990s, Calvin Klein underwear models, with their great abs, were getting more publicity than Tom Cruise and Tom Selleck combined. Today, Janet Jackson and Britney Spears have pushed the envelope even further.

The bottom line for both arms and abdominals goes back to the law of supply and demand. What is scarce and difficult to achieve is valuable—and not only valuable but attractive.

Arms and abdominals! Please make mine strong and muscular.

If that is what you wish for, then Bowflex furnishes a dynamic group of exercises for both these body parts. My recommended, best Bowflex exercises for the arms and the abdominals are as follows:

ARMS

Standing Biceps Curl

Lying Biceps Curl

Lying Triceps Extension

Seated Triceps Extension

Triceps Pushdown

Reverse Curl

ABDOMINALS

Seated Abdominal Crunch

Seated Oblique Crunch

STANDING BICEPS CURL

TARGETED BODY PART: FRONT OF UPPER ARMS

JOINT MOTION: ELBOW FLEXION

MUSCLE WORKED: BICEPS

PULLEY POSITION: WIDE

STARTING POSITION

- Remove bench and set aside.
- Straddle rail and face Power Rods.
- Grasp handles with palms facing forward and stand.
- Keep elbows at sides with wrists straight throughout movement.

ACTION

- Curl handles smoothly in arcs toward shoulders. Do not move upper arms.
- Pause in contracted position.
- Lower handles slowly to starting position.
- Repeat for required repetitions.

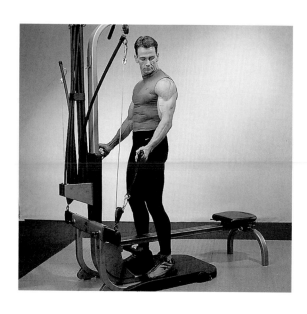 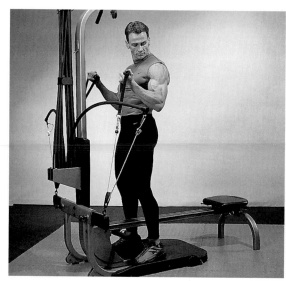

TRAINING TIPS

- Keep repetitions strict. Do not lean shoulders forward or backward. • Pause briefly at top, but do not pause at bottom.
- Grip handles moderately.

LYING BICEPS CURL

TARGETED BODY PART: FRONT OF UPPER ARMS

JOINT MOTION: ELBOW FLEXION

MUSCLE WORKED: BICEPS

PULLEY POSITION: WIDE

STARTING POSITION

- Sit on bench facing Power Rods.
- Grasp handles with palms up.
- Lie back on bench with arms straight and feet flat on platform.

ACTION

- Curl handles smoothly in arcs toward shoulders.
- Pause in contracted position.
- Return slowly to starting position.
- Repeat for required repetitions.

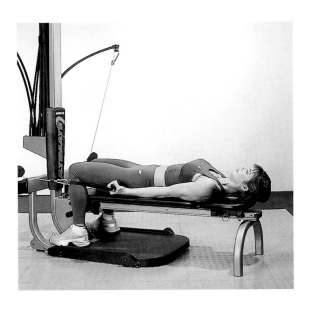 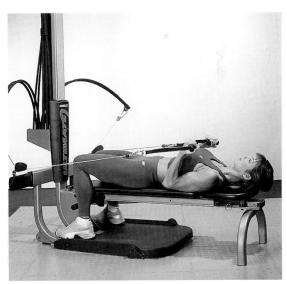

TRAINING TIPS

- Do not move upper arms during exercise. Keep them stable. • Keep face relaxed, especially during final repetitions.
- Breathe freely.

LYING TRICEPS EXTENSION

TARGETED BODY PART: BACK OF UPPER ARMS

JOINT MOTION: ELBOW EXTENSION

MUSCLE WORKED: TRICEPS

PULLEY POSITION: NARROW

STARTING POSITION

- Lie on back with head toward Power Rods.
- Reach overhead and grasp handles with palms up.
- Bring handles to shoulders with elbows bent.
- Move upper arms to sides for stability. Make sure feet are flat on floor.

ACTION

- Extend elbows smoothly.
- Continue until arms are straight and handles are near hips.
- Pause in contracted position.
- Return slowly to starting position.
- Repeat for required repetitions.

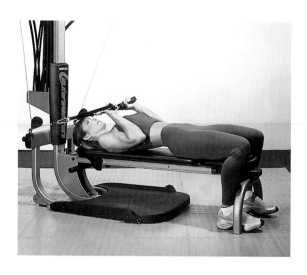
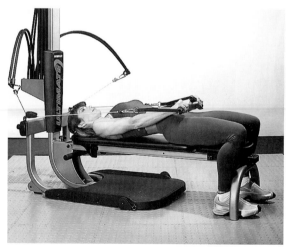

TRAINING TIPS

- Be smooth in all repetitions. • Keep upper arms stationary. • Avoid moving shoulders, head, and feet.

SEATED TRICEPS EXTENSION

TARGETED BODY PART: BACK OF UPPER ARMS

JOINT MOTION: ELBOW EXTENSION

MUSCLE WORKED: TRICEPS

PULLEY POSITION: NARROW

STARTING POSITION

- Adjust seat to 45-degree position and sit facing away from Power Rods.
- Grasp handles and bring to shoulders.
- Position feet flat on floor.
- Straighten arms to front and bring handles together with thumbs nearly touching.

ACTION

- Lower handles slowly to forehead while keeping upper arms stationary.
- Press handles in arc overhead.
- Repeat for required repetitions.

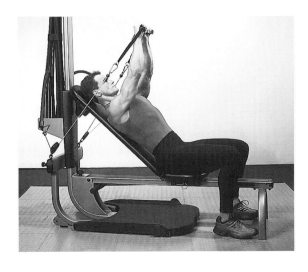 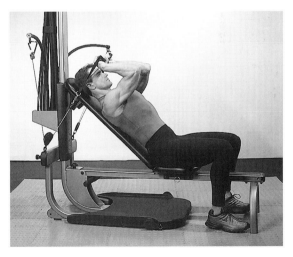

TRAINING TIPS

- Practice using a moderate resistance at first. This is a difficult exercise to master. • Stabilize torso by keeping shoulder blades pinched together during entire movement.

TRICEPS PUSHDOWN

TARGETED BODY PART: BACK OF UPPER ARMS

JOINT MOTION: ELBOW EXTENSION

MUSCLE WORKED: TRICEPS

PULLEY POSITION: NARROW

STARTING POSITION

- Remove bench and set aside.
- Straddle rail and face Power Rods.
- Use long lat bar or small T bar.
- Grasp bar with palms down.
- Position body so pulleys are approximately 12 inches in front of torso.
- Maintain upper arms at sides with elbows bent.
- Widen feet on platform, if necessary, and keep knees slightly bent throughout exercise.

ACTION

- Straighten arms smoothly by pushing bar in arc.
- Continue until bar is near front hips.
- Pause in contracted position.
- Return slowly to starting position.
- Repeat for required repetitions.

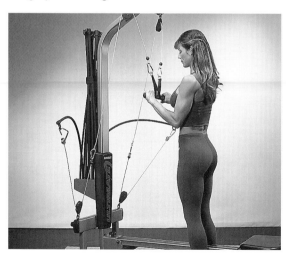 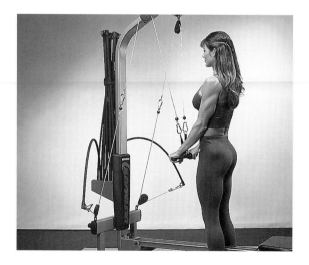

TRAINING TIPS

- Maintain good posture. Do not move shoulders up, down, forward, or backward. • Keep upper arms motionless.
- Maintain straight wrists throughout exercise.

REVERSE CURL

TARGETED BODY PART: FRONT UPPER ARMS AND FOREARMS

JOINT MOTION: ELBOW FLEXION (IN PRONATION)

MUSCLES WORKED: BRACHIALIS, BICEPS, BRACHIORADIALIS

PULLEY POSITION: WIDE

STARTING POSITION

- Remove bench and set aside.
- Straddle rail and face Power Rods.
- Grasp one handle and spread cuff. Slide hand through so pad rests on back of hand and tighten. Do same for other handle.
- Stand with palms down and arms straight.

ACTION

- Curl handles smoothly with palms down.
- Continue until handles are near shoulders.
- Pause in contracted position.
- Lower slowly to starting position.
- Repeat for required repetitions.

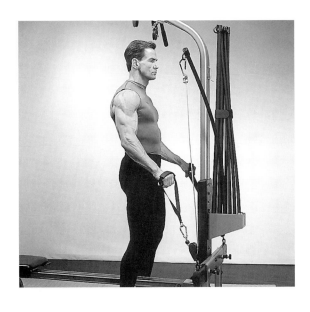 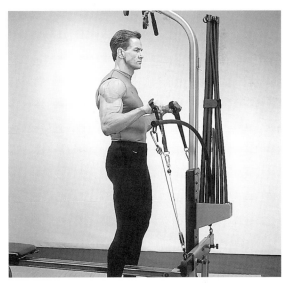

TRAINING TIPS

- Keep wrists straight during movement. • Do not move elbows forward or backward. • Maintain slow, smooth movements on all repetitions.

SEATED ABDOMINAL CRUNCH

TARGETED BODY PART: FRONT WAIST

JOINT MOTION: SPINAL FLEXION

MUSCLE WORKED: RECTUS ABDOMINIS

PULLEY POSITION: NARROW

STARTING POSITION

- Adjust bench to 45-degree position and sit facing away from Power Rods.
- Grasp handle, spread cuff, and slide entire arm through cuff until it is around shoulder. Do the same thing with other cuff and shoulder.
- Make sure cuffs are comfortably over front of both shoulders.
- Crisscross hands over cuffs or place near waist.
- Place feet securely on floor.

ACTION

- Tighten abdominals and smoothly move ribs toward hips. This is a short, focused motion.
- Pause in contracted position. When fully crunched, lower back should still be in contact with bench.
- Return slowly to starting position, but do not pause. Begin the next crunch immediately.
- Repeat for required repetitions.

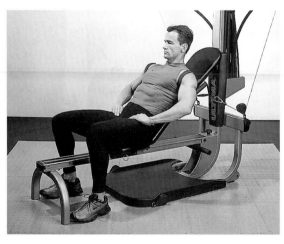 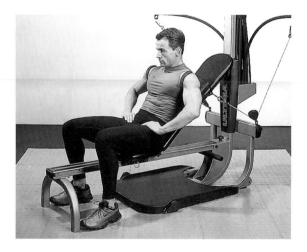

TRAINING TIPS

- Note: An assistant or workout partner can greatly help getting into starting position. • Do not lead with chin/head. Lead with ribs and let head follow. • Keep abdominal muscles tight throughout entire movement.

SEATED OBLIQUE CRUNCH

TARGETED BODY PART: FRONT AND SIDES OF WAIST

JOINT MOTION: SPINAL FLEXION WITH ROTATION

MUSCLES WORKED: RECTUS ABDOMINIS, EXTERNAL OBLIQUE, AND INTERNAL OBLIQUE

PULLEY POSITION: NARROW

STARTING POSITION

- Adjust bench to 45-degree position and sit facing away from Power Rods.
- Grasp one handle, spread cuff, and slide arm through cuff until it is around shoulder.
- Crisscross hands over shoulders or place near waist.
- Place feet securely on floor.

ACTION

- Tighten abdominals and smoothly move in a diagonal direction, from attached side toward opposite hip. Remember, this is a short, focused movement.
- Pause in contracted position. When fully crunched, lower back should still be in contact with bench.
- Return slowly to starting position, but do not pause. Begin next crunch immediately.
- Repeat for required repetitions.
- Switch sides and work other side in same manner.

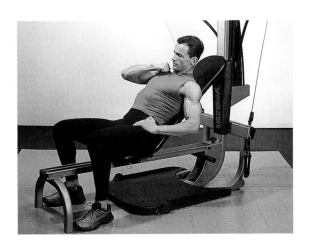 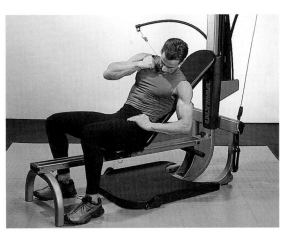

TRAINING TIPS

- Note: This is a one-sided version of the Seated Abdominal Crunch. No assistance is necessary. • Keep repetitions slow and controlled. • Lead with ribs, not head. • Do not hold breath.

9
BASIC TRAINING:

ROUTINES FOR BEGINNERS & INTERMEDIATES

THERE ARE MANY KINDS OF ROUTINES that you can perform with your Bowflex machine. In the *Owner's Manual and Fitness Guide*, routines are listed under the following headings: 20-minute better body workout, advanced general conditioning, bodybuilding three-day split, circuit training, aerobic circuit, and strength training. Some of the routines recommend that you perform more than one set. You can try any of these routines or others that you may have in mind. Before you do, however, let's review some basic guidelines.

As I mentioned in chapter 5, I'm a strong believer in doing one set per exercise, working from larger to smaller muscles, and performing twelve or fewer exercises per workout. Where did these beliefs come from? They came from my experience, spread over forty years, of personally training thousands and thousands of people on Nautilus equipment. Along the way, I also worked with many athletes on free weights and, since 1995, several hundred people on Bowflex. I also wrote about what I learned and observed in individual case studies or group studies and published that information in many magazines and books.

Publishing fitness information and recommendations can be a humbling experience. My peers in the field—nearly a thousand well-educated and experienced fitness professionals—provide constant criticism that forces me continually to reexamine the assumptions behind my work.

While working on this book, I've once again reexamined these assumptions. Consequently, I've determined that sometimes, *new* is better; other times, *old* is better.

The basics of strength training haven't changed much in the past thirty years. In fact, I explained them in an article I wrote for *Athletic Journal* in 1975. No, Bowflex didn't exist then. If it had, though, I would recommend almost the same type and style of routines I did in that article.

PLANNING A ROUTINE

Chapters 6, 7, and 8 describe and illustrate twenty-three Bowflex exercises. For easy reference, they are listed below.

LOWER BODY

Leg Curl

Leg Extension

Leg Press

Seated Leg Curl

Seated Calf Raise

BACK

Seated Row

Lying Lat Pulldown

Reverse Grip Pulldown

CHEST

Bench Press

Chest Fly

Incline Bench Press

Lying Shoulder Pullover

SHOULDERS

Standing Lateral Raise

Seated Shoulder Press

Shoulder Shrug

ARMS

Standing Biceps Curl

Lying Biceps Curl

Lying Triceps Extension

Seated Triceps Extension

Triceps Pushdown

Reverse Curl

ABDOMINALS

Seated Abdominal Crunch

Seated Oblique Crunch

Naturally, you wouldn't want to do all twenty-three exercises in a single routine. To do so, you would have to decrease the intensity, which is not an efficient way to build strength. The correct guideline is to select twelve or fewer exercises, separated into two to six exercises for your lower body and four to eight exercises for your upper body.

ROUTINES FOR BEGINNERS

A beginner is someone who is not familiar with strength training and has never used a Bowflex machine to train. With beginners, I recommend only six exercises initially. This eases the task of learning the exercises and reinforces good form.

After weeks 1 and 2, add two more exercises, then another two after weeks 3 and 4, and a final two after weeks 5 and 6. Thus, after only six weeks a beginner can perform up to twelve exercises in a workout.

One thing I've observed in more than forty years of strength training is that most beginners start with too many exercises in their initial routines and too much variety in their schedules. Doing so usually leads to poor results, low motivation, and a quick exit from the program.

Remember what I said in chapter 5 about the importance of understanding the basics? Hammer yourself with the fundamentals first. Learn good

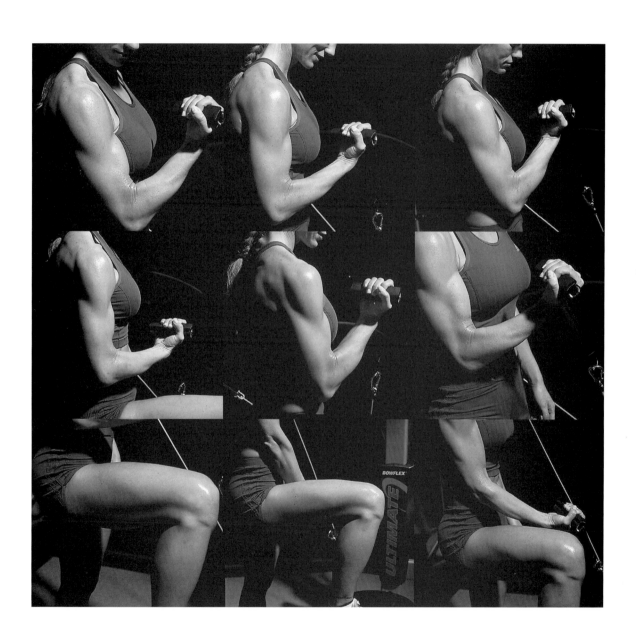

form—and practice, practice, practice—on the recommended six, eight, and ten basic Bowflex exercises over the first six weeks. It's the quality and not the quantity of exercise that's most important, especially during this critical time.

Six routines for beginners are included in this section. After the first routine, each workout is slightly longer and more complex than the one preceding it. It's a good idea to warm up before each workout with some seated rowing. Again, one set of 8 to 12 repetitions is the rule on all exercises, and your goal is to repeat the appropriate routine for three nonconsecutive days per week.

ROUTINE 1 FOR WEEKS 1 AND 2

1. Leg Curl

2. Leg Extension

3. Bench Press

4. Seated Row

5. Lying Shoulder Pullover

6. Seated Abdominal Crunch

If your Bowflex machine doesn't have a Leg Extension/Leg Curl Attachment, substitute the Seated Leg Curl for the Leg Curl, and the Leg Press for the Leg Extension.

ROUTINE 2 FOR WEEKS 3 AND 4

1. Leg Curl

2. Leg Extension

3. Seated Calf Raise*

4. Bench Press

5. Seated Row

6. Lying Shoulder Pullover

7. Shoulder Shrug*

8. Seated Abdominal Crunch

*New exercise

The Seated Calf Raise and the Shoulder Shrug improve the thoroughness of Routine 2. Focus on perfecting your form on each repetition of each exercise.

ROUTINE 3 FOR WEEKS 5 AND 6

1. Leg Curl

2. Leg Extension

3. Seated Calf Raise

4. Bench Press

5. Seated Row

6. Lying Shoulder Pullover

7. Shoulder Shrug

8. Lying Triceps Extension*

9. Standing Biceps Curl*

10. Seated Abdominal Crunch

*New exercise

Routine 3 increases the burden on the upper arms with the addition of the Lying Triceps Extension and the Standing Biceps Curl. You'll feel the effects on your upper arms almost immediately.

ROUTINE 4 FOR WEEKS 7 AND 8

1. Leg Curl

2. Leg Extension

3. Leg Press*

4. Seated Calf Raise

5. Bench Press

6. Seated Row

7. Standing Lateral Raise*

8. Lying Shoulder Pullover

9. Shoulder Shrug

10. Lying Triceps Extension

11. Standing Biceps Curl

12. Seated Abdominal Crunch

*New exercise

Routine 4 adds the Leg Press and the Standing Lateral Raise. Since you've completed six weeks of progressive training, you should be able to tackle a twelve-exercise routine that taxes both your muscular strength and your cardiovascular endurance. Your goal is to make it through the routine in less than 30 minutes.

ROUTINE 5 FOR WEEKS 9 AND 10

1. Leg Curl

2. Leg Extension

3. Leg Press

4. Seated Calf Raise

5. Chest Fly*

6. Reverse Grip Pulldown*

7. Standing Lateral Raise

8. Lying Shoulder Pullover

9. Shoulder Shrug

10. Lying Triceps Extension

11. Standing Biceps Curl

12. Seated Oblique Crunch*

*New exercise

During Routine 5, you eliminate the Bench Press, Seated Row, and Seated Abdominal Crunch. In their place, you add the Chest Fly, Reverse Grip Pulldown, and Seated Oblique Crunch. This variety should spur your motivation. If you don't have a Lat Tower, substitute the Lying Lat Pulldown for the Reverse Grip Pulldown.

ROUTINE 6 FOR WEEKS 11 AND 12

1. Leg Press

2. Leg Extension

3. Leg Curl

4. Seated Calf Raise

5. Chest Fly

6. Reverse Grip Pulldown

7. Seated Shoulder Press*

8. Lying Biceps Curl*

9. Triceps Pushdown*

10. Standing Lateral Raise

11. Reverse Curl*

12. Seated Oblique Crunch

*New exercise

During Routine 6 there's a change in the order of the Lower-Body Exercises. The Leg Press is first, rather than third. You'll find that you're stronger in the Leg Press but slightly weaker in the Leg Exten-

sion and Leg Curl. In the same light, you now do the Leg Extension before the Leg Curl. Also, you drop four exercises: Lying Shoulder Pullover, Shoulder Shrug, Lying Triceps Extension, and Standing Biceps Curl. You add the Seated Shoulder Press, Lying Biceps Curl, Triceps Pushdown, and Reverse Curl. If you don't have a Lat Tower, apply the Seated Triceps Extension instead of the Triceps Pushdown.

INTERMEDIATE ROUTINES

An intermediate is someone who has trained on the beginning Bowflex routines for at least 12 weeks or someone who is already experienced in using Bowflex or other strength-training machines. Of course, the primary consideration is that you feel confident with your Bowflex machine. Increased strength breeds confidence—and you should be significantly stronger, by as much as 50 percent, in most of your exercises as an intermediate.

If you feel you still need some practice on the Bowflex exercises, then I'd suggest repeating Routines 4, 5, and 6—which will require another six weeks. Doing so will increase your strength, understanding, and confidence—and prepare you for the intermediate routines.

There are six intermediate routines included in this section. Once again, I recommend that you stick with each routine for two weeks, repeating each routine three nonconsecutive days per week.

PUSH-AND-PULL ROUTINE

1. Leg Extension

2. Leg Curl

3. Leg Press

4. Lying Shoulder Pullover

5. Bench Press

6. Shoulder Shrug

7. Seated Shoulder Press

8. Standing Biceps Curl

9. Triceps Pushdown

10. Reverse Grip Pulldown

11. Seated Abdominal Crunch

As the names imply, pushing and pulling exercises alternate a pushing exercise with a pulling exercise. Generally, pushing and pulling facilitates recovery because working both sides of a joint—agonist and antagonist muscles one after the other—is more efficient at creating blood flow to the targeted body parts.

PRE-EXHAUSTION ROUTINE

1. Leg Extension

2. Leg Press

3. Seated Calf Raise

4. Leg Curl

5. Chest Fly, immediately followed by

6. Bench Press

7. Lying Shoulder Pullover, immediately followed by

8. Reverse Grip Pulldown

9. Standing Lateral Raise, immediately followed by

10. Seated Shoulder Press

This routine pairs a single-joint exercise with a multiple-joint exercise. If paired correctly, the single-joint movement isolates a specific muscle, then the multiple-joint exercise brings into action surrounding muscles to force the isolated muscle to a deeper level of fatigue, which is good.

All multiple-joint exercises—such as the Bench Press, Seated Shoulder Press, and Reverse Grip Pulldown—have a weak link. The smaller, weaker muscles involved in the movement usually tire before significant growth stimulation occurs in the stronger muscles. Pre-exhaustion solves this problem. In the

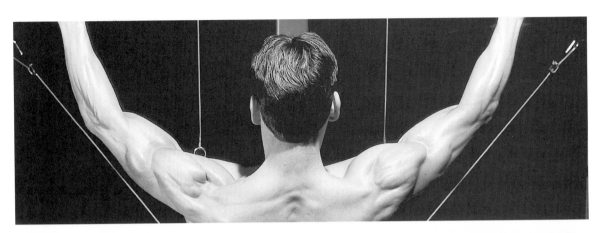

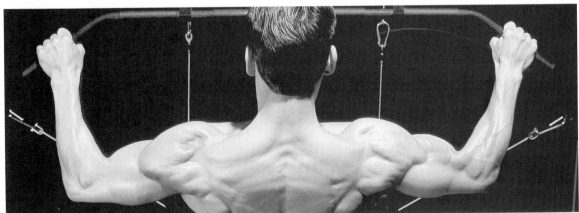

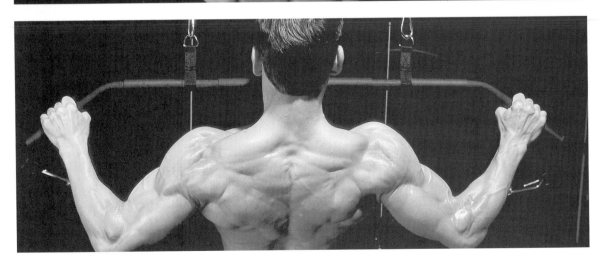

Bowflex Bench Press, for example, your triceps tire before your larger pectorals do. You can combat this weak link by pre-exhausting your pectorals.

First, do 8 to 12 repetitions of the Chest Fly. The Chest Fly works your pectoralis major muscles without much involvement of your triceps. Next, immediately do the Bench Press for as many repetitions as possible. When you reach a point of failure on the Bench Press, it will not be because your triceps fatigued before your pectorals were worked properly. When you fail, it will be because your pectorals are exhausted. Your pectorals will now be stimulated to grow larger and stronger.

The same concept applies with the Standing Lateral Raise and Seated Shoulder Press, the Lying Shoulder Pullover and Reverse Grip Pulldown, and the other paired exercises.

Important: For pre-exhaustion to work most effectively, you must move quickly between the paired exercises. Ten seconds between exercises is about average, but 5 seconds is much better. In fact, having a workout partner nearby to help you quickly change the bench and Power Rods will be a great help.

SUPERSLOW ROUTINE

1. Leg Extension

2. Leg Curl

3. Lying Shoulder Pullover

4. Bench Press

5. Reverse Grip Pulldown

6. Triceps Pushdown

7. Lying Biceps Curl

SuperSlow is a trademarked training system developed by Ken Hutchins. The primary difference of SuperSlow is in the way a repetition is performed: 10 seconds to lift and 10 seconds to lower. In other words, each repetition requires 20 seconds as opposed to the standard 6 seconds.

Bowflex, because of the Power Rods that increase their resistance as they bend, is not ideal for SuperSlow repetitions. SuperSlow is best performed on machines that supply a resistance curve that decreases in the contracted position. Nevertheless, you can still get a nice feel from SuperSlow repetitions on the Bowflex exercises. And performing SuperSlow repetitions certainly helps to improve your exercise form and focus.

Several guidelines are necessary for doing the SuperSlow Routine. First, I've decreased the number of exercises from ten to twelve to six to eight. Second, reduce your Power Rod resistance by approximately

25 to 30 percent of what you would normally do for 10 repetitions on each exercise. Third, cut your number of repetitions in half. Instead of using 8 to 12, apply 4 to 6 repetitions.

NO-TIME-TO-TRAIN ROUTINE

1. Leg Press

2. Reverse Grip Pulldown

3. Bench Press

4. Seated Abdominal Crunch

This routine is for the very busy person. You can get in and out of your home gym in 10 minutes and still get a fairly complete workout. Try it if you are pressed for time.

CHANGE-OF-PACE ROUTINE

1. Standing Biceps Curl

2. Lying Triceps Extension

3. Seated Abdominal Crunch

4. Bench Press

5. Leg Press

6. Seated Calf Raise

7. Overhead Press

8. Shoulder Shrug

9. Reverse Grip Pulldown

10. Leg Curl

11. Leg Extension

If you're looking for a routine that's a little different, this one goes against working the largest muscles first and the smallest muscles last. In fact, you start with the upper arms and finish with the thighs. It offers a nice change of pace for several weeks.

LOWER-BODY/UPPER-BODY SPLIT

Lower-Body Routine

1. Leg Curl

2. Leg Press

3. Lying Shoulder Pullover

4. Leg Extension

5. Leg Press

6. Lying Shoulder Pullover

7. Seated Calf Raise

8. Seated Oblique Crunch

Upper-Body Routine

1. Shoulder Shrug

2. Standing Lateral Raise

3. Seated Shoulder Press

4. Reverse Grip Pulldown

5. Seated Triceps Extension

6. Lying Biceps Curl

7. Bench Press

8. Reverse Curl

This split routine trains your lower body on one day and your upper body the next. Instead of a whole-body workout three times a week, with the lower-body/upper-body split, you're dividing it in half and training six times a week. Remember in chapter 5 I emphasized that rest and recovery ability was important for sustained strength-training success? Well, split routines and six-day-a-week training can tax your recovery ability in a major way and lead to overtraining.

Since I've been asked repeatedly by trainees for help in organizing a split routine for the lower and upper body, I've developed the exercise groupings in this routine. Here are my comments on how to apply them, if you must, to avoid overtraining:

• Perform the lower-body/upper-body split routine four times per week instead of six times per week. For example, train your lower body on Monday and Thursday and your upper body on Tuesday and Friday. Rest on Wednesday, Saturday, and Sunday.

• Include the abdominals in the lower body.

• Do two sets of the Leg Press. A set immediately after the Leg Curl emphasizes the hamstrings; doing them after the Leg Extension hits the quadriceps.

• Perform a set of the Lying Shoulder Pullover immediately after each set of the Leg Press. Since your breathing rate is at a high level during and after the Leg Press, the Pullover helps to expand your rib cage.

YOUR GOAL: DOUBLE YOUR STRENGTH

The Beginning and the Intermediate Routines will give you a broad selection of workouts for at least six months. Your goal at the end of six months should be to double your strength on the basic exercises that you started in Routine 1. Go back and examine your workout chart from week 1. If you did 60 pounds of resistance for 10 repetitions on the Leg Curl during the first week, then your goal is to do 120 pounds for 10 repetitions. If you've trained hard over the last six months, then you should be able to accomplish this goal. The same applies to the Leg Extension, Seated Row, Bench Press, Lying Shoulder Pullover, and Seated Abdominal Crunch.

Devote a workout to testing yourself on each of these six Bowflex exercises. If you are not quite twice as strong on one or more of the exercises, then don't fret. You will soon be at this level and, no doubt, will have made substantial progress toward this goal. Return to Routine 1 and focus on getting stronger in these exercises. In several weeks you should be at this double-your-strength level.

After you've doubled your strength, it's time to progress to the Advanced Techniques. That's the subject of the next chapter.

So grab your workout gear and let's get ready to rumble with those Power Rods!

10

ADVANCED TECHNIQUES:

BREAKDOWNS, DOUBLE PRE-EXHAUSTION, & NEGATIVES

"ALL THE BODYBUILDERS I KNOW back home," a friend of mine from England once said, "skip the beginning and intermediate routines and head straight to the advanced workouts. Even a complete novice likes to think of himself as being advanced."

That friend was Chris Lund, who is a world-famous photographer of bodybuilders. In 1983, Lund and I teamed up to produce *The Nautilus Advanced Body-building Book*. The book's success prompted us to put together three more courses—*Super High-Intensity Bodybuilding, Massive Muscles in 10 Weeks*, and *BIG*—for advanced trainees.

In concept, Lund is right. Many people, especially bodybuilders, tend to want only the hard-core, most intense material. But as Ilanon Moon and Arthur Jones, my greatest teachers, would say: "The advanced is not much good—in fact, it can be detrimental—unless you first understand the fundamentals."

So please don't get into this chapter unless you understand—and know how to apply—the fundamentals. That means you need to have mastered the Beginning and Intermediate Routines, spending at least six months training correctly with them on your Bowflex machine.

Don't make the mistake, *even if you are a serious bodybuilder*, of assuming you can bypass the basics. You can't.

Besides the length of time that a person has been strength training, the primary difference between beginners and advanced trainees is something called *inroad*. An advanced trainee frequently wants to make a deeper inroad into his starting level of strength.

A DEEPER INROAD

What happens on a typical set of 10 repetitions of a Bowflex exercise? *Inroad* plays an important role in the answer, as the following example explains.

Let's say a trainee performs 1 repetition with 100 pounds of Power Rods on the Standing Biceps Curl. A second repetition is not possible. In fact, he barely accomplished the first one. So let's call 100 pounds his starting level of strength.

Research shows that instead of performing a series of 1-repetition sets, he will get much better muscle-building results if he reduces the resistance by 20 percent and performs as many repetitions as possible. So he puts 80 pounds on the Power Rods and grasps the handles. Eighty pounds feels easy at first, because he is 100-pounds strong. But with each succeeding repetition, he makes a deeper inroad into his starting level of strength. By the 10th repetition, his temporary level of strength is 81 pounds—just barely enough to lift 80 pounds of resistance. Then, the trainee fails on the 11th repetition.

Thus, after 10 repetitions with 80 pounds on the Standing Biceps Curl, the trainee has reduced his starting level of strength to 79 pounds or less. In doing 10 repetitions, he has made a 21 percent or greater inroad into his starting level of strength, an optimum level if the trainee is a beginner or intermediate.

But what would happen if, rather than the trainee failing on the 11th repetition, the resistance was reduced to 60 pounds? With 20 pounds less, the trainee could continue to perform repetitions until his biceps strength was reduced below the resistance on the Power Rods—until his muscles failed. That technique is called *breakdowns*.

Besides breakdowns, two other advanced techniques—*double pre-exhaustion* and *negatives*—are described in this chapter. All three of these techniques make deeper inroads into a person's starting level of strength. Breakdowns and double pre-exhaustion are best performed with the help of an assistant. A section on each follows.

BREAKDOWNS

The correct way to do breakdowns is as follows:

• Decide beforehand by how much you are going to break down the Power Rods. A 20-percent reduction is suggested.

• Instruct your assistant to stand behind the Power Rods.

• Perform your normal set to failure. Stay in the exercise position without dropping the handles.

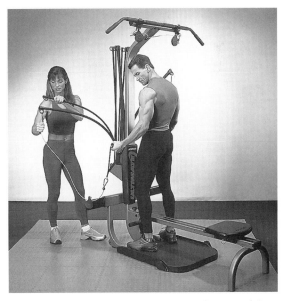

Breakdowns: As an example, during your first set of the Standing Biceps Curl, on the last repetition, it's your assistant's job to decrease the Power Rods by 10 percent. After a quick transition, continue performing the exercise.

• Have your assistant quickly readjust the Power Rods—first one side, then the other—to the predetermined breakdown resistance.

• Continue doing repetitions slowly and smoothly.

Your goal is to do half as many repetitions during the breakdown set as you did during the first set. Try to do 1 more repetition in each succeeding breakdown workout. Record the number of repetitions on your workout log. When you can do 12 repetitions in the first set and 6 repetitions in the breakdown set, up the resistance on the first set.

For best results, breakdowns should almost be one extended set rather than two separate sets. Thus, your assistant must readjust the Power Rods quickly—while still being careful with the adjustment process.

Breakdowns are most effective when they are used on your upper body. They work well on deltoids, pectorals, biceps, triceps, and forearms.

DOUBLE PRE-EXHAUSTION

Normal pre-exhaustion is performed when a single-joint exercise for a specific muscle is followed by a related multiple-joint movement. The multiple-joint movement brings into action the surrounding muscles to force the previously exhausted muscle to a deeper level of fatigue.

For example, the Seated Triceps Extension on a Bowflex machine isolates your triceps, and the Bench Press involves your pectorals and deltoids, as well as your triceps. Perform the Seated Triceps Extension and the Bench Press back to back, with no rest between them, and you'll feel a deep level of exhaustion within your triceps. As a result, you will stimulate new growth.

Double pre-exhaustion for the triceps goes a step further. Instead of doing two exercises back to back, you perform three in a row. For example, you can do two single-joint movements back to back and follow them with a multiple-joint exercise. Or you can do a multiple-joint movement, then a single-joint movement, and finally a multiple-joint exercise.

Here are a few recommended double pre-exhaustion cycles for various muscles. Perform each group of three with minimum rest in between.

TRICEPS

1. Incline Bench Press

2. Seated Triceps Extension

3. Bench Press

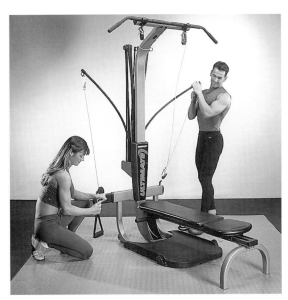

Double Pre-Exhaustion: Between the three exercises, you and your assistant must quickly make appropriate adjustments to the Power Rods, pulley positions, hand grips, cables, and lat tower.

1. Triceps Pushdown

2. Seated Triceps Extension

3. Bench Press

BICEPS

1. Lying Biceps Curl

2. Standing Biceps Curl

3. Reverse Grip Pulldown

1. Reverse Grip Pulldown

2. Standing Biceps Curl

3. Seated Row

CHEST

1. Incline Bench Press

2. Chest Fly

3. Bench Press

SHOULDERS

1. Shoulder Shrug

2. Standing Lateral Raise

3. Seated Shoulder Press

BACK

1. Reverse Grip Pulldown

2. Lying Lat Pulldown

3. Seated Row

All of these Double Pre-Exhaustion cycles are guaranteed to tax the targeted muscle group to the ultimate—if you can maintain your focus and endure the muscle-burning pain.

NEGATIVES

In weight-training circles, a repetition is divided into two parts—the positive and the negative. The lifting phase is called positive; the lowering phase is called negative. Up is positive; down is negative. A typical repetition, therefore, includes both lifting and lowering, both positive and negative.

As you know, a Bowflex machine does not involve the lifting and lowering of metal plates or weight stacks. Power Rods, which bend and extend, supply the resistance. And these Power Rods furnish both positive and negative phases. Bending Power Rods furnish positive resistance and extending Power Rods provide negative resistance. Bending is positive and extending is negative.

In the 1970s, research that separated and compared positive and negative resistance found the following:

• Negative strength is 40 percent greater than positive strength. In other words, if you can lift 200 pounds maximally, then you can lower, under control, 280 pounds.

• Since you can lower more than you can lift, negative repetitions allow you to make a greater inroad into your starting level of strength.

• Negative repetitions tend to make the targeted muscles and attachments very sore over the following forty-eight hours.

Anyone who has trained with negative repetitions on a barbell soon discovers a major problem: you have to have a couple of strong training partners who are willing to do all the lifting for you after you concentrate on lowering the barbell. After several workouts of them doing the lifting and you doing the lowering, they may not want to show up—at least, not on time. Ideally, you would have a machine that could do the lifting for you.

That's exactly what Arthur Jones of Nautilus Sports/Medical Industries accomplished in 1972. He built prototypes of several motor-driven machines that did the positive lifting for a trainee. These machines eventually proved to be too large and expensive to produce. Several smaller versions without motors were manufactured, however. They worked by incorporating a leg-press apparatus into an upper-body machine.

Thus, a trainee could use his legs to lift the movement arm into the contracted position, where he transferred the load to his shoulders, chest, or upper arms for the negative phase. In other words, he did the positive with his legs and the negative with a specific upper-body muscle group.

Since lower-body strength exceeds upper-body strength, individuals could provide a negative workout for their upper bodies—without the assistance of a partner. These machines worked moderately well for the advanced trainee, but they were discontinued after five years.

Another one of Jones's ideas about negative resistance proved to be more fruitful and is applicable to the Bowflex Leg Curl/Leg Extension Attachment. What he determined was that on almost any leg-curl or leg-extension machine with a fused movement arm, you can lift the movement arm with both legs, and lower it with only one leg. This lift-with-two, lower-with-one concept allows you a chance to stress the negative on your quadriceps and hamstrings. Jones called such training *negative accentuated*.

Here's how negative-accentuated training works with the Bowflex Leg Extension.

• Note amount of resistance you do normally for 10 repetitions with both legs.

• Take 70 percent of that resistance. For example, if you do 100 pounds for 10 repetitions, then put 70 pounds of Power Rods on machine.

• Assume your normal leg-extension starting position.

• Lift resistance with both legs to contracted position.

• Pause at top and transfer load from two legs to one leg. Keep loaded leg straight. It should not bend or bobble during transfer. If it does bend or bobble, reduce resistance.

• Move unloaded leg slightly away from pad.

• Lower slowly in 8 seconds with one leg by bending knee.

• Lift movement arm back to top with both legs.

• Pause, transfer, and lower in 8 seconds—this time with other leg.

• Up with two, down with one.

• Up with two, down with the other.

• Continue until you can no longer get to contracted position with both legs.

If the resistance is selected correctly, you should reach a point of momentary muscular failure at about the 11th or 12th repetition. When you can perform 12 repetitions, you should increase the resistance by 10 pounds. A properly performed set of negative-accentuated Leg Extensions will consist of eight to twelve lifting or positive movements, plus four to six lowering or negative movements performed by each leg.

The Bowflex Leg Curl works equally well as a negative-accentuated exercise. Do it in the same way as the Leg Extension. Up two, down one. Up two, down

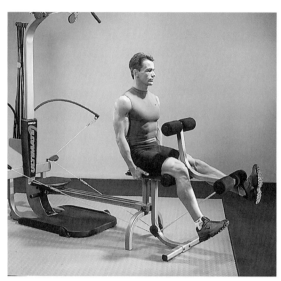

Negatives: With the Leg Extension/Leg Curl attachment, you can accentuate the negative by lifting the resistance with both legs and lowering with only one leg.

with the other. Remember, try to do each negative very slowly in 8 seconds.

Two other Bowflex exercises work fairly well in a negative-accentuated fashion. They are the Leg Press and the Seated Calf Raise. They both require the Leg Press Belt Attachment. Select a light resistance at first and experiment with the transference of the load from both legs to one leg. The best way is to simply lift the unloaded leg slightly off the footrest or upright pulley frame as you perform the lowering. Keep the unloaded foot and leg nearby, just in case you need a little help. Once you get the feel of both movements, the exercise should proceed smoothly.

ADVANCED ROUTINES

Successful Advanced Routines adhere to four guidelines:

• Use eight exercises per routine. Remember, more exercise is not better. Harder exercise is your goal.

• Limit an advanced technique in a routine to four exercises or less.

• Reduce the training frequency from six times in two weeks to five times in two weeks. Sometimes, with strong individuals, four times in two weeks is recommended.

• Apply each Advanced Routine for five consecutive workouts. Try all the Advanced Routines in this fashion. You may return to a favorite routine after two months.

Each of my Advanced Routines is listed below, with comments that follow. *Note:* Perform the bracketed exercises with minimal rest in between.

BREAKDOWN ROUTINE, UPPER ARMS

1. Leg Curl

2. Leg Extension

3. Chest Fly

4. Lying Lat Pulldown

5. Standing Biceps Curl, break down Power Rods by 20 percent

6. Standing Biceps Curl

7. Lying Triceps Extension, break down Power Rods by 20 percent

8. Lying Triceps Extension

You'll need an assistant to stand behind the Power Rods and carefully reduce the resistance after exercises 5 and 7. Sure, you can drop the handles and do it yourself, but the overall effect is not the same. Try to begin exercise 6 and exercise 8 in fewer than 3 seconds after finishing the previous ones.

BREAKDOWN ROUTINE, SHOULDERS

1. Leg Press

2. Seated Calf Raise

3. Standing Lateral Raise, break down Power Rods by 20 percent

4. Standing Lateral Raise

5. Reverse Grip Pulldown

6. Seated Shoulder Press, break down Power Rods by 20 percent

7. Seated Shoulder Press

8. Seated Oblique Crunch

A breakdown on Standing Lateral Raise, done properly, really hits the middle deltoid. You'll probably be unable to raise your arms after these back-to-back sets. The Reverse Grip Pulldown gives your shoulders a brief chance to recover before they're attacked from a different angle with the Seated Shoulder Press. Once again, you'll need someone to break down the Power Rods after the first set.

DOUBLE PRE-EXHAUSTION ROUTINE, BACK

1. Leg Curl

2. Leg Extension

3. Reverse Grip Pulldown

4. Lying Lat Pulldown

5. Seated Row

6. Incline Press

7. Shoulder Shrug

8. Seated Triceps Extension

This Double Pre-Exhaustion Routine for the back involves two multiple-joint exercises separated by a single-joint movement. You and your assistant need to practice several times all the adjustments that are necessary to perform these three movements one after the other. Remember, the quicker you can move between these three exercises, the better as far as your targeted muscles are concerned.

DOUBLE PRE-EXHAUSTION ROUTINE, TRICEPS

1. Leg Extension

2. Leg Press

3. Seated Calf Raise

4. Triceps Pushdown

5. Seated Triceps Extension

6. Bench Press

7. Standing Biceps Curl

8. Seated Abdominal Crunch

This Double Pre-Exhaustion Routine for the triceps involves two single-joint movements followed by a multiple-joint exercise. You'll need to hustle between exercise 4 and exercise 5, since there's a change of the cables as well as the bench. Do your best to keep the focus on the back of your arms.

NEGATIVE-ACCENTUATED ROUTINE,

THIGHS AND CALVES

1. Leg Curl, Negative Accentuated (NA)

2. Leg Extension (NA)

3. Seated Calf Raise (NA)

4. Bench Press

5. Reverse Grip Pulldown

6. Standing Lateral Raise

7. Standing Biceps Curl

8. Triceps Pushdown

On the three leg exercises, perform 70 percent of your normal resistance in the negative-accentuated style. Up with two legs; down with one. Up with two; down with the other. Perform the other five exercises in a normal manner.

NEGATIVE-ACCENTUATED ROUTINE,

THIGHS AND HIPS

1. Leg Curl or Leg Extension (NA)

2. Leg Press (NA)

3. Seated Row

4. Seated Shoulder Press

5. Shoulder Shrug

6. Incline Press

7. Lying Biceps Curl

8. Seated Abdominal Crunch

On exercise 1, you may choose between the Leg Curl and the Leg Extension. Or you can alternate between them. The Leg Extension before the Leg Press does make a greater inroad into your pressing strength, so you'll need to adjust the resistance on the negative-accentuated Leg Press accordingly.

MORE POWER TO YOU!

That's a wrap on Advanced Techniques and the routines that include them. Your arsenal is now packed with productive information. All you have to do is plan, aim, and fire. You're sure to be on target.

The power is yours to get the results you've always wanted. Take advantage of this power now.

While you're resting and relaxing between workouts, you'll want to explore Part III. Part III's eight chapters discuss the science behind what's happening to your body. Yes, you want more muscle and less fat, but there's more to the process than you've probably imagined.

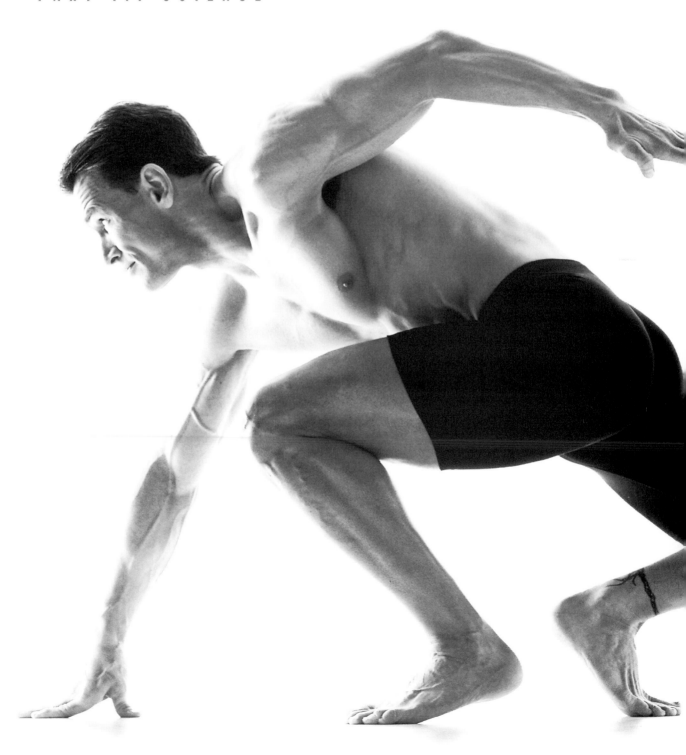

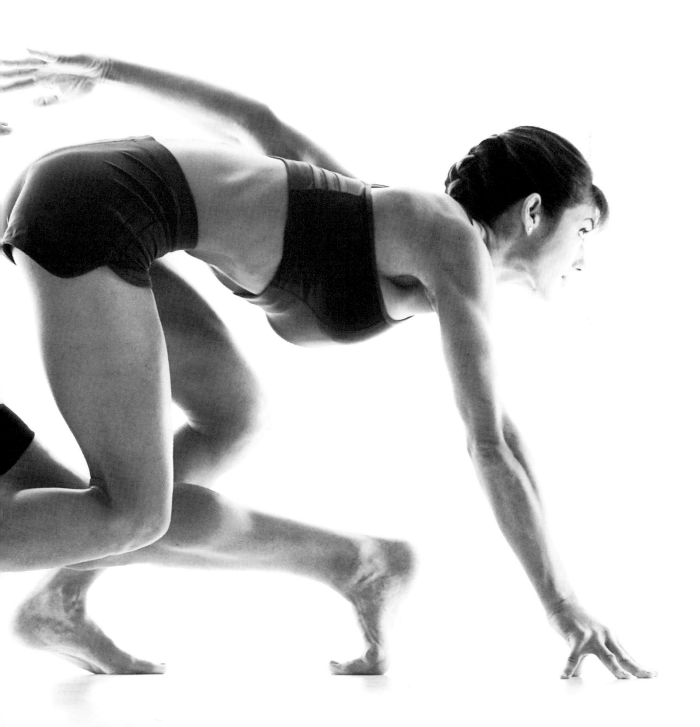

11
MUSCLE:
HARD TO GET, EASY TO LOSE

MUSCLE HAS BEEN OUR ENGINE, our means of movement, since the beginning of our time on Earth. With muscle we run, kick, jump, throw, and swim. With it we lift heavy objects and thread tiny needles, operate chain saws and manipulate keyboards.

Our muscle varies only slightly from that found throughout the animal kingdom. From ants to whales, bats to yaks, caterpillars to zebras—muscle ambulates, propels, and steers us all. Our muscles aren't as strong as an ant's or as enduring as a whale's. But on both accounts, they come close to nature's best.

As a testament to our strength and endurance, the Great Pyramid of Egypt and the Great Wall of China were both built primarily by human muscle. The Great Pyramid is composed of more than 2 million blocks of limestone, each weighing from 2 to 70 tons. You could build thirty Empire State Buildings with its masonry. The Great Wall of China, which is from 15 to 30 feet thick and 25 feet tall, stretches about 1,500 miles across northern China. It's one of the few things that can be seen clearly while orbiting Earth.

The Great Pyramid was constructed 4,600 years ago, and the Great Wall of China was largely completed 2,200 years ago. Both these projects took lifetimes to complete and nearly lifelong muscle power from tens of thousands of people.

THE ADVANTAGES OF STRONG MUSCLES

History abounds with extraordinary feats of muscular strength. Sometimes unappreciated, however, is the fact that strong muscles also:

Protect you from injury. Strengthen your muscles and you also toughen your tendons, ligaments, and bones, which equals greater structural integrity for your body.

Govern metabolism. Larger, stronger muscles rev up your metabolism significantly.

Look attractive. If you are lean, muscles make up from 30 to 50 percent of your body weight. Greek and Roman sculpture idealized body leanness and muscularity for its simple beauty.

Burn calories. Muscles are richly supplied with energy carried by blood through veins and capillaries. They require a steady flow of calories to keep functioning. Add a pound of muscle to your body and your body needs an extra 37.5 calories per day to keep it alive.

Support overlying fat and skin. There are 434 skeletal muscles throughout your body. These muscles are the primary foundation for shaping your physique beneath the layers of fat and skin.

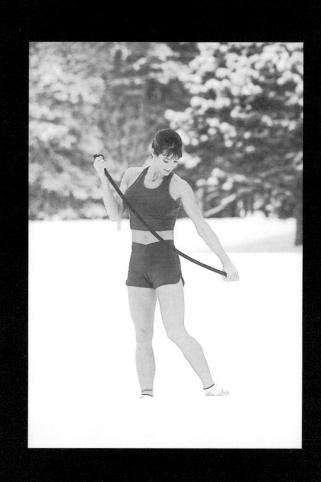

Allow you to work your cardiovascular system. Since your muscles contract and produce movement, they are the only things that generate sustained action for working your heart in a progressive manner.

HOW MUSCLES GROW LARGER AND STRONGER

Muscular growth, very simply, is a two-step process. First, stimulate the muscle with an overload. Second, permit the stimulated muscle to grow by providing adequate rest. Remember, muscle grows during rest, not during exercise. Chapter 5 discusses the exercising and resting guidelines that are necessary for the most efficient muscular growth.

Beneath this two-step process, however, is the science of the muscular-growth process. Each muscle consists of thousands of cylindrical fibers. These fibers divide into hundreds of thousands of myofibrils, which separate into millions of filaments of actin and myosin. When a muscle grows, the actin and myosin filaments initially increase of size and/or number. This increases the circumference of the myofibrils, which in turn expands the cylindrical muscle fibers. As a result, muscle fibers grow wider, not longer—and they increase in size, not number. This process is called *hypertrophy*.

Another growth process is called *hyperplasia*. Hyperplasia is when muscle fibers split, which increases the total number of fibers. This method of muscular growth occurs primarily in cats and other smaller mammals. There is little evidence that it occurs in healthy humans. Hypertrophy is the way that human muscles grow.

The opposite of hypertrophy is atrophy. *Atrophy* is when muscle fibers shrink or waste away from lack of use. There are plenty of physical problems that are related to atrophy.

ATROPHY RESEARCH

Use it or lose it. That's the popular concept related to muscle that is taught in most physical education courses in the United States. The concept certainly applies to strength training. If you work harder this week than last week, your muscles grow slightly stronger. If you don't work as hard this week as you did the previous week, then a small amount of atrophy, or shrinkage, occurs.

A lot of the basic research on muscle atrophy was done by Dr. Gilbert Forbes of the Rochester School of Medicine. I first met Forbes during a 1975 West Point study, which I discussed in chapter 3. He helped with the body-fat calculations of the cadets.

At that time, Forbes was in the process of analyzing longitudinal data on the body composition of men and women he had monitored for several decades. His full report was published in *Human Biology* in 1976. Basically, what he discovered was that average men and women between the ages of twenty and fifty, who do not strength train, lose half a pound of muscle per year. Eight ounces per year translates into slightly more than $^{22}/_{100}$ of an ounce per day, which seems insignificant. And it probably would be, if not for the cumulative effect. (Interestingly, much of Forbe's original research has been reinforced with the latest body-composition technology by scientists at the Nutrition, Exercise, Physiology, and Sarcopenia Laboratory at Tufts University in Boston.)

Bit by bit, little by little, ounce by ounce, things add up. After a decade, it's 5 pounds. After thirty years, it's 15 pounds.

A loss of 15 pounds of muscle is nothing to laugh about. The next time you're at the supermarket, spend some time in the meat department. Pick up a 5-pound roast. Imagine holding three 5-pounders. That's approximately the space in your body that 15 pounds of your muscle occupies. Of course, atrophy is not selective, it happens throughout your body, from all of your muscle areas.

Perhaps two of the pounds shrink from each thigh, another pound from each buttocks, a couple of pounds from your back, chest, and shoulders, and finally, a half pound from each arm and each calf, and the remaining several pounds from around your lower back, midsection, and neck.

If that scenario is not enough to make you want to go and work out, then the next facts will for sure.

Forbes also found that while average men and women are losing muscle ounce by ounce, they are gaining fat at triple the rate. That fat gain amounts to 1½ pounds each year, or 15 pounds per decade. That's a 45-pound fat gain over thirty years.

Fat tissue is approximately 20 percent less dense than muscle, so it takes up 20 percent more space. Next time you're at the supermarket, look at a 40-pound sack of dog food. That's how much space the fat takes up on your body. Get the picture?

THE EFFECT ON METABOLISM

Your resting metabolism is the number of calories your body requires to operate in a relaxed state. Your brain and internal organs—your heart, lungs, liver, and kidneys—demand a lot of energy. But it's your muscles, which comprise from 30 to 50 percent of a lean person's body weight, that use the most energy.

Lose a pound of muscle through atrophy and your resting metabolic rate goes down approximately 37.5 calories per day. Add a pound through strength training and your rate goes up by the same number.

A pound of fat tissue inside the human body also has a metabolic rate: approximately 2 calories per day. Muscle is thus 18.75 times as metabolically active as the same amount of fat.

FIBER TYPES: THE SKINNY ON SLOW AND FAST

Muscular contraction starts in the brain. Nerve cells, called neurons, send signals to the appropriate muscle fibers. A neuron and the muscle fibers that it controls are collectively known as a motor unit.

Motor units and muscle fibers are generally classified as slow twitch, type I, or fast twitch, type II. Type II is further divided into type IIa and type IIb. *Slow* and *fast* refer to the way a muscle tires.

Slow-twitch fibers are used when the activity requires low force for extended periods of time. Fast-twitch fibers join the action when you need great force, but they tire quickly.

It's important to understand that motor units and muscle fibers are always recruited in a set order: from small to large, from slow to fast. Regardless of the speed of the activity, fast-twitch fibers are never used unless the slow-twitch fibers have been recruited first. If the force needs of an activity are low, you will use only slow-twitch fibers, even if it's a fast movement like swatting a fly. If the force requirements are high, as in seeing how much you can bench press one time, you'll be using both your slow-twitch and fast-twitch fibers, even if you're moving slowly.

Arthur Jones, in the early 1990s, tested thousands of volunteers on a work-capacity test involving a computerized MedX Lumbar-Spine Machine. This test, among other things, allowed him to measure the fatigue characteristics—slow or fast—for the muscles that were involved in lumbar extension. Here's what he found:

- Almost 80 percent of the volunteers had a similar combination of slow-twitch and fast-twitch fibers (such as 40–60, 50–50, and 60–40). These volunteers performed best in strength training by using 8 to 12 repetitions.
- Ten percent of the volunteers had predominantly slow-twitch fibers. They performed best by employing higher repetitions: 16 to 20.
- Ten percent of the volunteers had predominantly fast-twitch fibers. They performed best with lower repetitions: 4 to 6.

It's fairly well known that as adults age they have a harder and harder time shedding their excessive fat. The reason: a decrease in metabolism.

Long-term metabolic studies reveal that an average individual experiences a 0.5 percent reduction in resting metabolic rate each year between twenty and fifty years of age. The gradual wasting away of muscle is primarily responsible for the metabolic slowdown.

Atrophy breaks down muscle into its constituent compounds, which are removed by the bloodstream. Muscle fibers, as they atrophy, actually lose their fluids and become smaller, weaker, and less supportive.

- Specific training does not change slow-twitch fibers to fast-twitch fibers or vice versa. Whatever a person's ratio, it's genetically determined and cannot be altered.

Occasionally, Jones would test a person who was extremely slow twitch or extremely fast twitch. The slow-twitch individual would be abnormally weak on the strength portion, but very enduring on the work-capacity part. On the other hand, the fast-twitch person would be abnormally strong, with little capacity for endurance.

After testing a dozen or so of each of the extreme-type individuals, Jones got to where he could pick them out of a large crowd without testing them. Why was this possible? Because radical slow-twitch individuals and radical fast-twitch persons have recognizable looks to their bodies.

Extremely slow-twitch individuals are tall, thin, and narrow-bodied with stringy muscles. The African athletes who are so successful at long-distance running are good examples of this, as are the vast majority of people who win ultra-endurance events.

Extremely fast-twitch people are strongly built, broad shouldered, and muscular, especially in the hands and arms. Athletes in this category who you might recognize are Mark McGwire (baseball), Dick Butkus (football), and Shaquille O'Neal (basketball), as well as the actor Michael Clarke Duncan.

By the way, according to *The Sporting News*, Shaquille O'Neal is the biggest athlete in major professional sports—not counting sumo wrestling or horse racing. In May of 2002, at a height of 7 feet 1 inch, Shaq weighed 382 pounds.

"The extremes at both ends are true genetic freaks," Arthur Jones says, and he uses *freaks* in an admiring sense. "They look like ten-carat diamonds in a handful of dirt. Those in the middle—and that includes most of us—are simply average. And they look like—well, average—average dirt!"

Well said from a man who is certainly anything but average.

The continued loss of muscle may manifest itself in physical ailments such as lower-back pain, bothersome knees and shoulders, arthritis, or even heart disease. From there, it's often a steady downward spiral.

A BOWFLEX CHALLENGE

Your body doesn't have to get caught up in this downward spiral. With Bowflex strength training, you can put a stop to the regression and actually reverse the process. You can rebuild atrophied muscle and, perhaps, grow your muscles larger and stronger than they've ever been.

No, it won't be easy, especially if you're over forty years of age. But it will be well worth it, as thousands and thousands of Bowflex believers will testify.

Besides building your muscle, that fat around your belly, hips, and thighs must be studied, analyzed, and—if it proves to be excessive—aggressively attacked. The next chapter deals with that.

12
FAT:

EASY TO GET, HARD TO LOSE

THE NEWS ABOUT FAT—THAT STUFF that clings so diligently around your belly, hips, and thighs—is not good. Since the year 2000, major wire services have reported the following.

Per capita, consumption of food in the United States increased by about 8 percent from 1990 to 2000, according to the Department of Agriculture. That translates to approximately 140 pounds of extra food per year per person. The primary reasons: Americans are eating out more, the servings are bigger, and the meals are consumed faster.

The United States is now the fattest nation on Earth, according to experts from the American Dietetic Association. The Russians used to be ranked number one, closely followed by the Germans. In the late 1990s, the United States was elevated to first place. If Americans keep on eating the way we do now, by 2030, theoretically, almost everyone in the United States will be obese.

The cost of treating obesity-related diseases, according to the National Institutes of Health, totals $52 billion annually. When indirect costs, such as lost productivity, are added in, the sum approaches $100 billion.

"Some 300,000 Americans a year die from illnesses caused or worsened by obesity," says Dr. David Satcher, a former U.S. surgeon general.

Obesity is joining and even surpassing malnutrition as a dietary concern throughout the world. Data from the United Nations agencies indicate 1.1 billion people get too few calories each day to ward off hunger. At least 1.1 billion or more people take in too many calories. In fact, according to Philip James, chairman of the International Obesity Task Force, as reported in *USA Today* (March 17, 2003), the number of obese people worldwide may be as high as 1.7 billion.

In China, for example, the proportion of overweight men has tripled in the past eight years, notes Dr. Barry Popkin of the University of North Carolina.

Food manufacturers in the United States compete fiercely for consumer dollars, spending $30 billion annually on advertising. "They want people to eat when they're not hungry," says Dr. Marion Nestle of New York University, "and keep eating when they're full." Large portions—such as supersized fries, 64-ounce soft drinks, and muffins as big as a cantaloupe—are the way they do that. "We are so programmed to eat everything in front of us," Nestle continues from an interview in *USA Today*. "Eating is fun, and not eating is not fun."

Parade, the Sunday newspaper magazine, in its annual issue (November 11, 2001), "What America Eats," reports Americans want it all: trimmer waistlines, faster foods, and tastier desserts. More than 33 percent of adults are dieting, 70 percent are "trying to cut fat," while eating an average of three desserts a week. Pizza is the favorite takeout meal and the number one food we couldn't live without if stranded on a desert island. Chocolate is number two. Chips are the number one choice for between-meal munching. Interestingly, pizza, chocolate, and chips are usually loaded with fat—the very thing most people are trying to cut down on!

THE *WHY* OF BODY FAT

If excessive fat on the body (or obesity, which some experts define as being 5 percent or more above the average fatness according to sex and age) is becoming such a health problem throughout the world, you might be wondering how and why it evolved. A brief history lesson is necessary.

When the first humans started migrating out of Africa more than 100,000 years ago, living was extremely hard. Snow and ice were often part of the climate, and humans had to adapt to the cold or die.

Fat storage was one of the first modes of adaptation. Body fat provided warmth, energy, stamina, and even aided successful reproduction. Thin people were inclined to die out, while those who were fatter tended to mate more successfully and survive.

Prehistoric men and women soon started to observe that those who thoroughly engorged themselves during times of feast tended to get fatter than those who did not. Gorging probably became a much-prized endeavor for the strongest men, and for the women they relished. You should realize that there was probably no one at that time who was even close to being obese. *Getting fatter* meant adding 4 or 5 pounds, or perhaps 6 or 7 pounds at the most. A little bit of fat still goes a long way, and back then it probably lasted even longer.

While living past age twenty-five was unlikely for most hunter-gatherers, another 5 pounds of fat, especially from a woman's point of view, might mean a pregnancy, a baby, and perhaps another year of life. Once again, extra body fat greatly increased a person's probability of survival. Thus, over hundreds of generations a preference for fatness, as opposed to leanness, was bred into the genes of humankind.

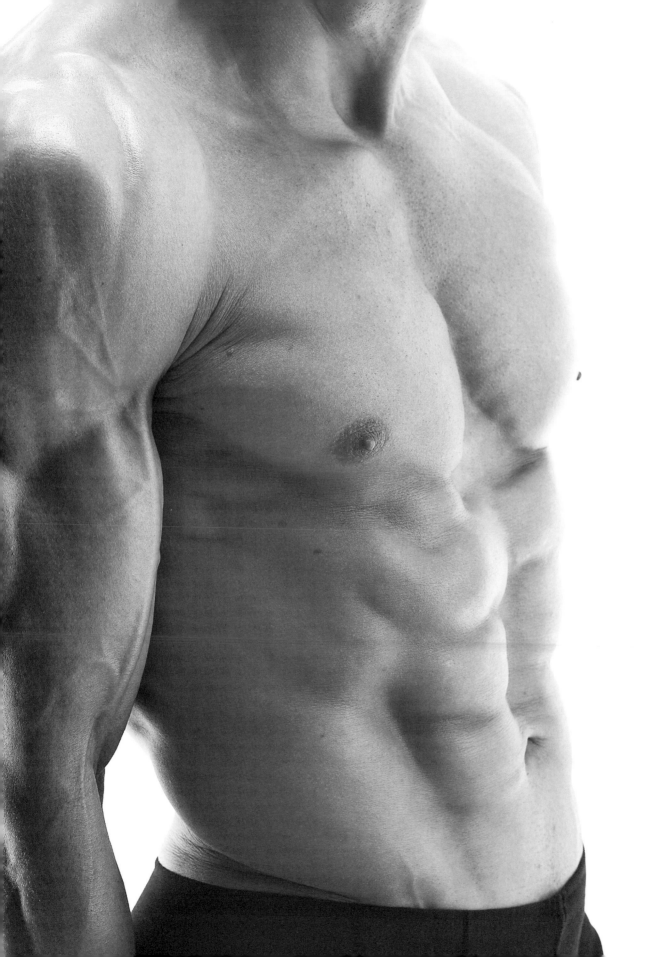

Even though times have changed greatly, the bias for fatness thrives in today's society. Why? Because it was only 12,000 years ago that the last Ice Age, where winters lasted ten months at a stretch, finally waned in northern Europe—a mere second or two on the evolutionary time clock. Try as we may, we can't get around a confrontation with those pesky fat cells. The best thing to do is to understand them, and then deal with them.

CHARACTERISTICS OF FAT CELLS

To understand fat cells you have to know their characteristics.

Consistency. At body temperature, fat is a thick, oily liquid that has a slight yellowish tint. It feels semisolid in your bulges because the walls of the cells keep it in place.

Chemistry. The liquid inside each fat cell is composed of 79 percent lipids, 15 percent water, and 6 percent proteins. The high concentration of lipids is the reason fat is such a potent source of calories. An ounce of fat contains 218.75 calories, which is almost six times as much as the same amount of muscle tissue. Since there are 16 ounces in a pound, one pound of fat contains 3,500 calories.

Types. There are three kinds of fat cells. *Subcutaneous* cells lie in the layers directly under the skin. *Depot* cells are deposited in areas determined by your genetic makeup—usually either your stomach or hips and thighs. *Essential* fat cells surround many vital organs. Generally, 50 percent of fat is subcutaneous, 40 percent is depot, and 10 percent is essential. You can successfully shrink your subcutaneous and depot fat cells, but not your essential fat cells.

Size. When I say fat cells are small, I mean microscopically tiny—each cell is smaller than a pinhead. Muscle cells, or fibers, are cylindrical in shape. Fat cells are round or globular.

Number. You count fat cells not in thousands, not in millions, nor even tens of millions—but by the billions. Scientists have taken fat samples throughout the body and actually totaled them. Although this research is still in its infancy and depends on extrapolation, some interesting findings emerge. The numbers of fat cells vary greatly according to your genes. Numbers range from a low of 10 billion to a high of 250 billion. Obviously, a person with a minimum number of fat cells has a lower probability of being fat compared to a person with a high number of fat cells.

Gender differences. The average woman in the United States has approximately 42 billion fat cells. The average man has about 25 billion fat cells. Women have 68 percent more fat cells than men primarily because their bodies need it to conceive and bear children.

A necessity for reproduction. Women add fat during pregnancy. It provides the caloric reserve required during the stress of childbirth. Nature has arranged matters so that, even without another person to provision her, the mother and infant can survive, at least for a while, on the mother's fat stores. Research also reveals that adolescent girls must have a minimum amount of fat before they start to menstruate.

Different storage spots. Men have more frontal fat than women. The "potbelly" and "love handles" are almost entirely the problems of middle-aged men. Women tend to deposit their fat on their backsides, primarily over their hips and upper thighs, with some spreading to the middle of the upper back and triceps of the arms. Women's breasts are also composed of fat cells.

Versatility. Fat cells in your favorite storage spots resemble a microscopically small bubble bath (with a million bubbles) inside an inner tube, which has the capacity to inflate or deflate as required. The cells are grouped together with stringy intercellular glue and streaked with narrow filaments of connective tissues, blood vessels, and nerves. Each cell, or bubble, can inflate to three or four times its normal size or shrink to a fraction of its size, as fat is stored or burned.

Ability to increase. Approximately 90 percent of your fat cells were in place at your birth. Genetics plays a huge role in your future fatness or leanness. But you can create some fat cells (approximately 10 percent) later in life. The primary times are during your first year, during puberty, and during pregnancy. Once you create new fat cells, they are yours for life. You can shrink them, but without surgery you can't get rid of them.

MEASURING THE AMOUNT OF FAT ON YOUR BODY

How do you determine how much fat you have on your body? Stepping on a standard scale may offer some clues, but it doesn't measure fat alone. Measuring your waist may also reveal some interesting numbers, but it doesn't tell you exactly how much fat you have. Disrobing in front of a full-length mirror and jumping up and down for a few seconds can offer even more insightful hints about parts that jiggle and bounce. But you still don't know how much is actually fat. What's needed is a device that deals with body fat.

Several tools and techniques have been developed to do just that. These include calculations based on X rays, ultrasound waves, underwater weighing, electrical impedance, and skin fold thickness. Most of these methods require special equipment and expertise and can be expensive.

For more than thirty years, I've used the Lange Skinfold Caliper to measure folds of skin and fat in various areas of the body. The method I recommend for taking skin folds and in turn calculating the percentage of body fat comes from work done by William Baum, Michele Baum, and Peter Raven, which was reported in the *Research Quarterly for Exercise and Sport* in 1981. You can schedule a skin fold/fat assessment at your local YMCA, fitness center, or university exercise-science department.

Or you can look in back of the *Bowflex Owner's Manual and Fitness Guide* under "Measurements" and "Determining Your Body Fat" for all the how-to information, including the appropriate charts and graphs. If that's not convenient, you can get it online at www.Bowflex.com.

What is too fat, what is too lean, and what is just right? Proper use of the skin fold caliper supplies you with a percentage of body fat, which allows you to make those judgments. For example, the last group

PERCENT BODY FAT: HOW LOW SHOULD YOU GO?

What is the *ideal* percentage of body fat for men and for women? Naturally, it varies, depending on such things as age, height, occupation, goals, as well as genetics. But generally, when I work with average people, such as the group of 150 people from Gainesville, I encourage men to strive for the 12 percent level, and women to work toward 18 percent. Some can reach this goal and go lower, some can't. Nevertheless, it's an ideal to shoot for.

With athletes, and genetically gifted people, the levels are lower. In chapter 21, The Hard-Body Challenge, one of the five professional water-skiers, Gary Smith, got his body fat down to 3.4 percent. In my opinion, that was too low. Five percent would have been better for him and for most other male athletes. Of course, it's fairly easy to curb fat loss by upping your calorie intake and continuing until you replenish your body-fat stores.

With female athletes, the lower limit is 12 percent. Below that level the hormones do not function properly.

of people I worked with on a six-week fat-loss program in Gainesville, Florida, had the following before-and-after body-fat percentages:

	Before	After	Difference
Men (N=41), Percent body fat	27.3	17.9	9.4
Women (N=109), Percent body fat	33.7	26.1	7.7

From these numbers, you should be able to discern several salient points. First, men start with a lower average fat percentage than women: 27.3 versus 33.7. Second, men lose a greater percentage of fat than women: 9.4 versus 7.7. Most of these differences have to do with what I mentioned earlier: hormones and the ability to bear children. (*Note:* When I do skin fold measurements, I consider a person obese if body fat percentage is above 20 percent for men and 30 percent for women.)

SHRINKING THOSE FAT CELLS

You should understand by now that body fat is easy to get but hard to lose. There's still much to be learned about shrinking your fat cells. As a preview, in the next six chapters, I'll cover such topics as meal composition and size, food supplements, superhydration, sleep, and synergy. All of these offer a piece to the solution.

Next, in chapter 13, I'm going to share with you a related idea that might at first sound strange: *thermodynamics.* Such a word certainly looks impressive, doesn't it? Well, the concepts behind it are impressive too, as you'll see.

13
THERMODYNAMICS:
SOMETHING OLD & SOMETHING NEW

THERMODYNAMICS IS THE BRANCH of physics dealing with the reversible transformation of heat into other forms of energy. Interestingly, *reversible transformation of heat* can mean fat gain or fat loss. The step-by-step understanding of this concept, however, involves going back to the early 1500s, when adventurers on sailing vessels traveled the world.

SIXTEENTH-CENTURY OBSERVATIONS

Imagine a seaside café in the Dutch city of Amsterdam where explorers sit at tables to enjoy food and beverage—and to describe the various places they have visited and the peoples they have observed. There's little doubt that such things as geography, climate, and the physical qualities of the peoples they met would be important topics of discussion.

After many years of travel and numerous round-table discussions, the smartest explorers and the wisest listeners probably would have made the following summations:

• People who live near the equator are thin and lean.

• People who live near the equator have dark-colored hair and skin.

• People who live great distances from the equator are thick and fat.

• People who live great distances from the equator have light-colored hair and skin.

Useful information? Yes. But without having specific measurements and comparisons of the peoples and the places, it would be difficult to move past these simple observations. Three hundred years later, such data were collected and assembled by two men working independently of each other: Carl Bergmann, a biologist, and J. A. Allen, an anatomist.

BODY SIZE AND CLIMATE

Bergmann and Allen, in the mid-1800s, drew a strong connection between body size and climate. They determined that colder climates demanded that both humans and animals become bulkier and heavier.

For example, many of the largest sea and land mammals are found in the northernmost reaches of the Northern Hemisphere. Size and general bulkiness give the animal a significant thermal advantage in a cold climate. As an animal gains in size, the increase in its skin surface is smaller than the gain in its total bulk, which is beneficial when heat conservation is a concern.

Of course, the opposite is advantageous in hot climates. Long arms and legs increase the surface area dramatically, which is important for efficient heat loss.

The Masai people live in one of the hottest regions of Africa. At an average height of 6 feet for the men, they are among the tallest and longest-limbed people on Earth. Then there are the Lapps, who live mostly above the Arctic Circle in far northern Europe. The Lapps are extremely short-limbed. The men average just over 5 feet in height and the women average a mere 4 feet 6 inches.

In 1953, anthropologist D. F. Roberts studied some 220 adult populations from all parts of the globe. He confirmed that indeed people with higher body weights occur more frequently in cold regions and people with lower body weights reside more in warm regions of the world.

COLOR OF HAIR AND SKIN

In 1977, I remember being intrigued by the relationship between the color of hair/skin and geography when I read Anne Scott Beller's book *Fat and Thin: A Natural History of Obesity.* Beller noted that over centuries and centuries, populations adapt to their geographical locations. The predominant physical type within any given region will be one that is best suited to the climate. The odds of blond hair being found in a sunny climate are low. Fair-skinned people do not adjust well to hot, open environments unless they spend most of their time indoors. The gene pool in such a climate will contain few genes for blondness but many for dark skin and hair.

Conversely, in colder countries, children with light skin and hair are able to extract more vitamin D from sunlight than can their dark-haired brothers and sisters. Thus, it is the blonds who thrive. Over the centuries, colder areas of the world will tend to accumulate genes for blondness and genes for dark hair will gradually become scarce.

The more I studied Beller's book the more I could see a relationship between color of hair/skin and leanness/fatness. In other words, if you have dark hair and skin, your ancestors probably came from the warmer regions of the world—and you have a higher probability of having genes for leanness. If you have light hair and skin, your family tree likely goes back to the colder regions of the world—and you have a higher probability of having genes that promote fatness.

In chapter 12, I discussed the fact that human fat cells can vary tremendously in number from person to person. Genetics are the primary reason for this variation. Obviously, a person with a minimum number of fat cells has a lower probability of being obese compared to a person with a high number of fat cells.

EINSTEIN TO THE RESCUE

Thermodynamics offers some simple transitions to your goals—thanks to Dr. Albert Einstein. What Einstein, and other scientists, proved was that *energy can't be created or destroyed. It can only be transferred.* From a scientific point of view, body fat is heat energy and heat energy is best expressed in calories. Remember, there are 3,500 calories in one pound of fat.

Judging from all the phony fat-loss products that are advertised—and the people who buy them and keep buying them—this principle is difficult to grasp and easily misunderstood. Please bear with me as I try to explain it in plain English.

THREE WAYS
TO EMIT HEAT CALORIES

When you lose fat, it transfers out of your body as heat in three ways: through your skin, lungs, and urine. Most of your daily heat loss emerges through your skin, primarily through radiation. This shouldn't be surprising, especially if you relate back to Bergmann's and Allen's work concerning long limbs,

increased skin surface area, and more effective heat loss. Keeping your arms, legs, and head uncovered permits better radiation. While radiation is the primary way heat transfers from your skin, it also dissipates through conduction, convection, and evaporation.

Conduction is the transfer of calories through direct contact, usually with cold water or cold air. One tip I learned from talking with Olympic wrestlers is that shivering burns approximately three times as many calories as sweating. Too much shivering, however, is detrimental. What is desirable is an almost-shivering state. Some Olympic wrestlers, frantic to lose that last half-pound that would allow them to compete in a lighter weight classification, would ease themselves into a tub of cold water to induce an almost-shivering state. Thirty minutes in the cold water usually generated the necessary heat loss for them to make their weight classification.

When you add in the modest effect of convection and evaporation to the total, as much as 85 percent of your daily calorie loss is through the surface area of your skin.

You also eliminate heat calories through your lungs, which you can easily observe by breathing out forcefully on a cold day. Your lungs act as a bellows. Inhalation brings in oxygen-rich air, which is vital for

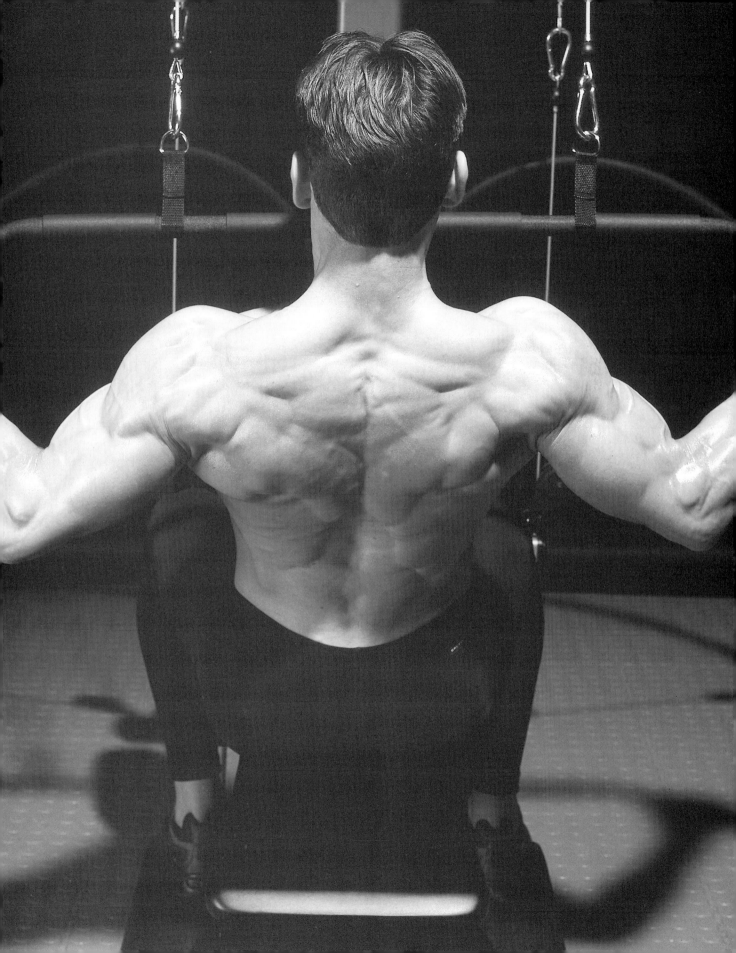

energy metabolism. Exhalation carries out oxygen-poor air and carbon dioxide. Approximately 10 percent of your daily heat-calorie loss occurs through your lungs.

The remaining 5 percent of your heat calories are eliminated through your urine. (*Note*: there's a small amount of heat in feces, but it's not significant unless you have diarrhea.) In chapter 16, you'll learn how you can dramatically increase your urine production, as well as heat loss, by drinking more water.

In summary, when you lose fat, it transfers from your body as heat through your lungs and urine, but primarily through your skin.

THE STRENGTH TRAINING TIE-IN

The efficiency of your skin at eliminating calories depends on the blood flow through it. Your skin, considering its entire surface area, is your body's largest organ. As a result, it's richly supplied with arteries, capillaries, and veins. As you shrink your subcutaneous fat, the vessels throughout your skin become more prominent. Competitive bodybuilders strive for that vascular, ripped look on their arms and legs, which makes them appear more muscular than they actually are.

The blood vessels of your skin enable this large surface area to function as a means of controlling the removal of calories, which thereby governs your body temperature. Here's the connection with proper strength training.

There is no better way to condition, revive, and rejuvenate your skin than to work the underlying muscles. With proper strength training you can isolate and work any part of your body—from the little muscles of your hands and feet to the large muscles of your thighs and chest—which directs blood to those targeted areas. This surging fluid brings nutrients and heat. The rising heat in the muscle must be released through your skin.

INTO THE ENVIRONMENT AND BACK

Lastly, when you lose fat, you transfer heat energy out of your body and into the environment. Once in the environment, it is available for use by other living organisms. These organisms use it and once again it is transferred, and the cycle continues endlessly.

Heat energy is everywhere. In basic biology we learn that the sun is our ultimate source of heat. The key to understanding solar energy, once again, is the transfer concept.

Humans have no way to take in this energy directly.

But plants can trap it by combining it with carbon dioxide and water. The product of this combination is a hydrated carbon, or carbohydrate. Only plants have the ability to grow by combining energy from the sun with the elements from air, soil, and water. Animals usually get their energy from consuming plants. Humans get energy from eating both plants and animals.

In simple terms, the sun transfers heat to plants, and plants transfer heat to animals. Both plants (through carbohydrates) and animals (through proteins and fats) transfer heat to humans. Humans transfer heat back to the environment, plants, and other animals.

HOW TO APPLY THERMODYNAMICS

Here are some practices related to thermodynamics that may assist you in losing heat calories:

• Dress in cooler colors and lighter fabrics at work, which won't trap the heat emanating from your body.

• Take off your coat sooner and keep it off longer. Select short sleeves more often.

• Drink cold water.

• Turn down the thermostat.

• Leave off the socks at home or go barefoot more frequently.

• Try to remain uncomfortably cool throughout the day and allow your skin's heating mechanism time to adjust.

• Strength train in a cooler environment if possible.

• Wear brief, well-ventilated clothing when you exercise.

• Minimize sweating by eliminating heat buildup.

• Avoid sauna, steam, and whirlpool baths, as they cause excessive heat accumulation.

• Sleep cooler.

• Wean yourself from electric blankets and flannel sheets in the winter.

THE NEW AND THE OLD

The reversible transformation of heat—that's the essence of thermodynamics. In losing body fat, for this biological phenomenon to make perfect sense, we have learned that you've got to factor geography and climate into the equation as well as your genetics. Being thorough—and realistic—will allow you to be more effective and satisfied with your efforts at losing fat.

May all your transfers, especially the fat ones, be worthwhile.

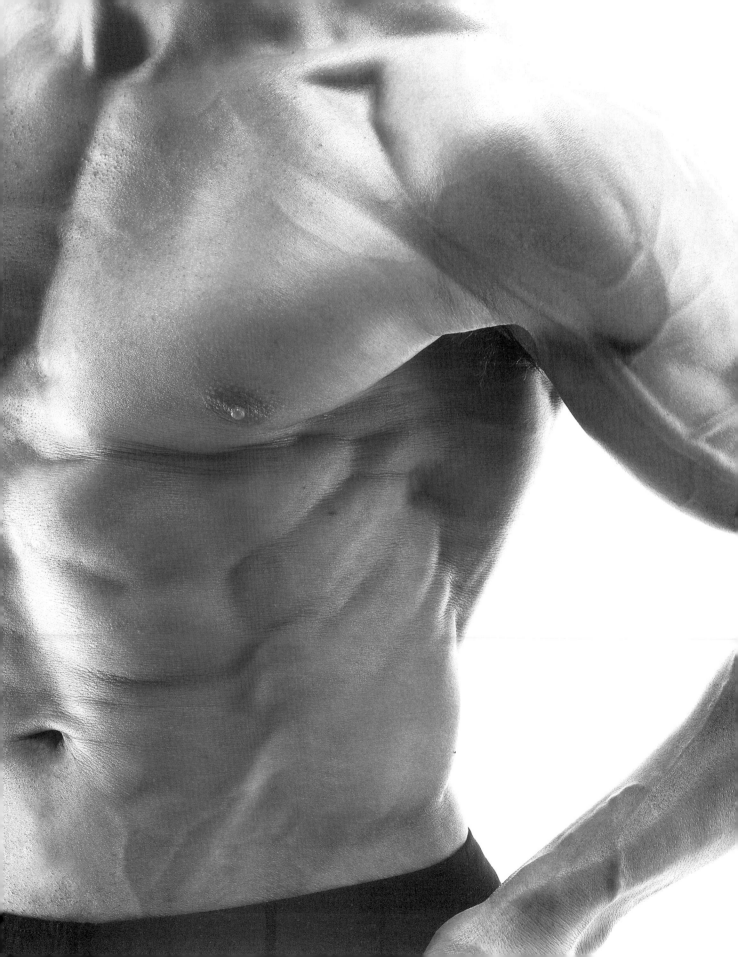

14

FAT-LOSS NUTRITION:

FUNDAMENTALS, SIMPLICITY, & DETAILS

Diets don't work!

How many times have you heard that over the past ten years? Probably a bunch—and for good reason.

According to *Consumer Reports* (June 2002), studies have shown that 95 percent of all dieters regain their lost weight and eventually add more pounds. Those are not very comforting statistics.

I'm here today, however, standing tall and looking you squarely in the eyes and saying: *Diets do work*—if they are grounded on certain fundamentals.

What are those fundamentals? They are the basics that are taught in university nutrition departments throughout the United States.

Oftentimes, the textbooks used in introductory nutrition courses are full of research findings and are not very exciting to read. Some students say they are boring. Compared to a lot of the best-selling eating plans, which are based on food faddism, these books don't get much attention.

It is not the intent of this chapter to provide a comprehensive view of basic nutrition. It would take far too many pages to do that. If you're interested, however, there are two introductory nutrition textbooks that I really like:

• *Nutrition: Concepts and Controversies* (ninth edition) by Frances S. Sizer and Eleanor N. Whitney, Wadsworth Publishing, 2003.

• *Understanding Nutrition* (ninth edition) by Eleanor N. Whitney and Sharon R. Rolfes, Wadsworth Publishing, 2001.

You can review these books on www.nutrition.wadsworth.com.

When I was in graduate school at Florida State University (1968–73), my first home was the exercise-science department. But my second home was the nutrition department. In fact, I completed two years of postdoctoral study under the direction of Dr. Harold E. Schendel, a professor of nutrition. Sharing the office with Schendel for several years was a young woman who had just completed a Ph.D. from Washington University in St. Louis. Her name was Eleanor Whitney.

Whitney had a great love for research and writing, and it certainly shows in her textbooks. I often talked to her about how to make the basics of good nutrition more available to the general population. She has done a great job with her books.

CRITERIA FOR A
SAFE, EFFECTIVE DIET

The number of weight-loss diets available in the United States is staggering. Researchers with the Health, Weight, and Stress program at Johns Hopkins University have collected and analyzed more than 29,000 methods for losing weight. Unfortunately, fewer than 6 percent of them were found to be effective or even safe.

From her research, Whitney has developed a list of seven criteria for a safe, effective diet. In question form, they are as follows:

• Does the diet provide a reasonable number of calories—an absolute minimum of 1,000 calories a day?

• Does it supply enough but not too much protein—at least the recommended 0.4 grams per pound of body weight but not more than twice that much?

• Does it supply enough fat for satiety but not too much—so that between 20 and 35 percent of the day's total calories come from fat?

• Does it supply enough carbohydrate per day to spare protein, so that you won't burn muscle tissue for energy, and enough to prevent ketosis—about 100 grams of carbohydrate for the average-sized person?

• Does it provide a balanced assortment of vitamins and minerals from whole-food sources in all of the basic food groups?

• Does it offer different foods every day so that you won't give up on the diet out of boredom?

• Does it consist of ordinary foods that are available in supermarkets at prices you can afford?

The diets that I've worked with and published over thirty years, including the ones in *The Bowflex Body Plan*, answer yes to all the criteria.

FROM COMPLEX TO SIMPLE

Today, however, I do a few things differently than I did fifteen years ago. As an example, in my book *The Nautilus Diet*, which was published in 1987, I had seventy-two recipes. Some of the recipes required more than 60 minutes of preparation and cooking time. In my most recent diet program, *A Flat Stomach ASAP* (1998), I have only two recipes. Both are for salads and require no more than 5 minutes to prepare.

Convenience and speed are even more of a priority today than they were in the 1980s. Thus, I sacrifice some of the variety that I used to recommend. In cut-

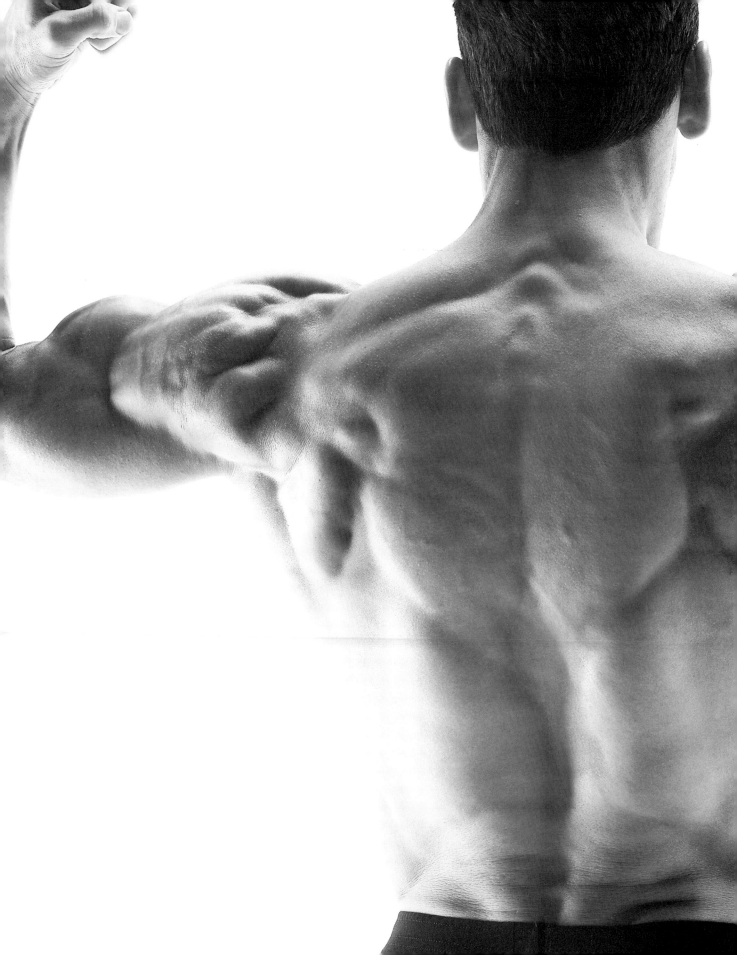

ting back on variety, I discovered some interesting behaviors:

• Dieters can eat the same breakfast each day for six weeks or longer without tiring of it.

• Dieters can eat the same lunch each day for six weeks without tiring of it. After six weeks they like a second choice for lunch.

• Approximately 75 percent of dieters can adapt to a meal-replacement shake mix for breakfast or lunch.

• Dieters like variety, at least three selections, for dinner each day.

• Approximately 90 percent of dieters like the convenience of frozen microwave meals for dinner.

• Dieters like between-meal snacks.

Next, by taking Whitney's criteria and combining them with my own findings, there are other salient details that merit discussion: meal composition, meal size, meal frequency, and calories per day.

MEAL COMPOSITION

A recent dietary survey found that the typical adult in the United States ate calories each day of the following composition: 46 percent from carbohydrates, 37 percent from fats, and 17 percent from proteins. Most nutritional scientists agree that Americans would be better off with more carbohydrates and less fats.

Most nutritional scientists also believe that carbohydrate-rich foods should make up at least 50 percent of a dieter's meals. I concur. In fact, after working with thousands of men and women who wanted to reduce fat, I've found that what worked best each day is the consumption of approximately 60 percent carbohydrates, 20 percent fats, and 20 percent proteins.

A 60:20:20 breakdown for each meal influences certain hormones, such as serotonin and cholecystokinin, which are important in producing satiation. Satiation is the process of feeling full and satisfied.

MEAL SIZE

Fat loss is aided by eating small meals. There's a thin line between a small meal and a medium meal. I draw that line at 400 calories for women and 500 calories for men.

Small meals facilitate fat loss because they result in small insulin responses. Insulin, a hormone produced in your pancreas, is the most powerful profat hormone and the primary promoter of fat preservation. It's a holdover from the Ice Age, when it was an advantage to be able to quickly store as much fat as possible. Eating larger meals stimulates more insulin production, which increases fat storage.

MEAL FREQUENCY

The goal is five or six small, evenly spaced meals a day. This means that no longer than three hours should elapse between eating episodes. Breakfast, lunch, and dinner are three eating episodes, and there are snacks at midmorning, midafternoon, and late at night. In this book, a snack of from 50 to 200 calories is classified as a small meal.

The sum of the five or six small meals, or the total number of calories that you consume each day, is the remaining factor of importance.

CALORIES PER DAY

In spite of what some people would have you believe, the laws of thermodynamics are constant. One gram of carbohydrate and one gram of protein each supply 4 calories, while one gram of fat contains 9 calories. And *all* calories from carbohydrates, proteins, and fats count against the total in losing fat. Once it is consumed, there is no way to weaken, discount, or bypass a food calorie. Bottom line is that you must consume fewer calories than you burn.

Your calorie intake, however, should not be too low, or your body may pull nutrients from your muscles and vital organs, and that's not desirable. The majority of the people I've worked with achieve optimum fat-loss results by adhering to daily calorie levels that range from 1,000 to 1,500. Women respond best to 1,000 to 1,300 calories a day. Men require slightly more, approximately 1,200 to 1,500 per day. A slight variation in the total number of daily calories on a weekly basis is also helpful.

MISTAKES, A GOOD TEACHER

"Success comes from good judgment. Good judgment comes from experience. Experience comes from bad judgment." That's a quote from Arthur Jones and I've heard him use it in his lectures.

In other words, many years of experience, the experience of making and correcting mistakes, teach a person how to appreciate both success and failure.

"We learn . . . when we learn," Jones continues, "only from our mistakes. Don't be afraid to make mistakes. But don't keep making them. Learn and move on.

"Be cautious, very cautious, of success. Success often serves to reinforce myth and superstition."

Jones is correct. Experience teaches caution, the same caution that is stressed throughout the science of nutrition.

As nutritional science progresses, there is the caution and tension between contradictory attitudes: an openness to new ideas, no matter how bizarre they may be, and a skeptical scrutiny of both new and old ideas. Remember those 29,000 fat-loss methods, with 94 percent of them classified as ineffective?

I've made mistakes. I've been skeptical. I've unlearned and relearned. And I'm still doing all of these. But along the way I've had some salient experiences about nutrition and fat loss, which I'm passing along to you in this book. Don't take my word for it, however. Be skeptical. Do your own research. Dig and then dig deeper.

THE BOTTOM LINE: RESULTS

The bottom line is that the methods and programs in *The Bowflex Body Plan* incorporate the latest research and they work. Do they work for everyone? Of course not. But they work for most people.

If you've had trouble losing fat and keeping it off in the past, I challenge you to understand and apply the guidelines in this book with precision. I believe you'll be surprised by the results.

I hope you'll give yourself a fair trial.

15

FOOD SUPPLEMENTS:

CONCEPTS TO CONSIDER

AT ONE TIME IN MY LIFE I FIRMLY BELIEVED that food supplements were good (I was a bodybuilder). At another time in my life I firmly believed that food supplements were bad (I was a scientist). Today, older and wiser, I recognize that indeed there is a place for a few food supplements.

One problem with dietary supplements is that their regulation falls into an odd category, sort of a large gray area between a food and a drug. As a result, the Food and Drug Administration allows manufacturers to make virtually any claim, other than that their product can prevent or cure a disease. Many supplements, especially those sold to bodybuilders, claim to do amazing things with virtually no science to back them up. In addition, testing has shown that many supplements do not consistently contain the active ingredients that are listed on the labels.

BACK TO GRADUATE SCHOOL

When I entered graduate school at Florida State University in 1968, I was heavily into bodybuilding. As a result, I consumed massive amounts of protein supplements each day. I took vitamin B_{12} for endurance, wheat germ oil for energy, garlic for purifying the blood, kelp tablets for muscle definition, and vitamin B_6 for strength. At the same time, I avoided white bread, carbonated drinks, ice cream, and most other carbohydrate-rich foods. I was convinced that this dietary program would help me become a superior athlete.

Where did I get these beliefs? The majority came from the bodybuilding magazines. According to these publications, most recent champions had followed such a program. I never questioned these concepts until I entered graduate school. In fact, I kept trying to find more concentrated protein supplements to be certain that I was consuming more than 300 grams of protein per day.

Remember Dr. Harold Schendel from the previous chapter? Well, Schendel was a guest lecturer in one of my exercise-science classes in the fall of 1968. All his basic nutrition facts seemed outdated to me and I was constantly interrupting his lecture with questions and comments that I thought were cutting edge. Schendel, a true scientist, was open-minded to my ideas, but he was also skeptical, especially since I had little evidence, other than my body, to back up what I believed. According to him, and he referenced the studies, an athlete did not require large amounts of vitamins, proteins, or any special foods.

Later that year, I spent many hours with Schendel discussing how various foods and eating habits might affect athletic performance and health in general. A major point of contention was supplements. I believed that athletes, especially bodybuilders, needed them in massive amounts. He thought supplements were unnecessary and even dangerous. Some of the discussions got fairly heated. Rather than argue, Schendel suggested that I experiment on myself as part of one of my graduate research projects.

All right, I thought to myself. I'll finally get a chance to prove that I know what I'm talking about.

A REVEALING EXPERIMENT

For two months, I kept precise records of my dietary intake, my energy expenditure, and my general well-being. My protein intake per day varied from 70 grams to 380 grams, most of which was obtained from a 90 percent protein powder. My calories averaged approximately 4,100 per day. All my urine was collected each day in two-gallon jugs—which is not an easy or fun thing to do—and analyzed to determine whether the protein I ate was being used by my body or merely broken down and excreted through my kidneys.

The results of the study were alarming to me. At the time, my body weight was 215 pounds. According to the Recommended Dietary Allowances (RDAs), my protein need was 77 grams per day. To my surprise, whenever I consumed more than this amount, the excess was excreted. My weight remained unchanged and I noted no difference in strength regardless of the amount of protein I consumed.

Furthermore, when I consumed more than the RDA of various vitamins and minerals, excess amounts of these substances were also excreted, rather than used, by my body.

I remember well when all the results were finally graphed on a chart. Afterward, I just walked around the nutrition laboratory in a daze for hours. Schendel was right. I was wrong, and I felt stupid and embarrassed.

Schendel saw it in a different light. "Now," he said, "you have the motivation to study the real science of food and nutrition. Let me help you."

"A single experience," Arthur Jones says, "can trigger a thought pattern that leads out of a blind alley . . . and having emerged into the light, you then have the opportunity to examine the involved factors."

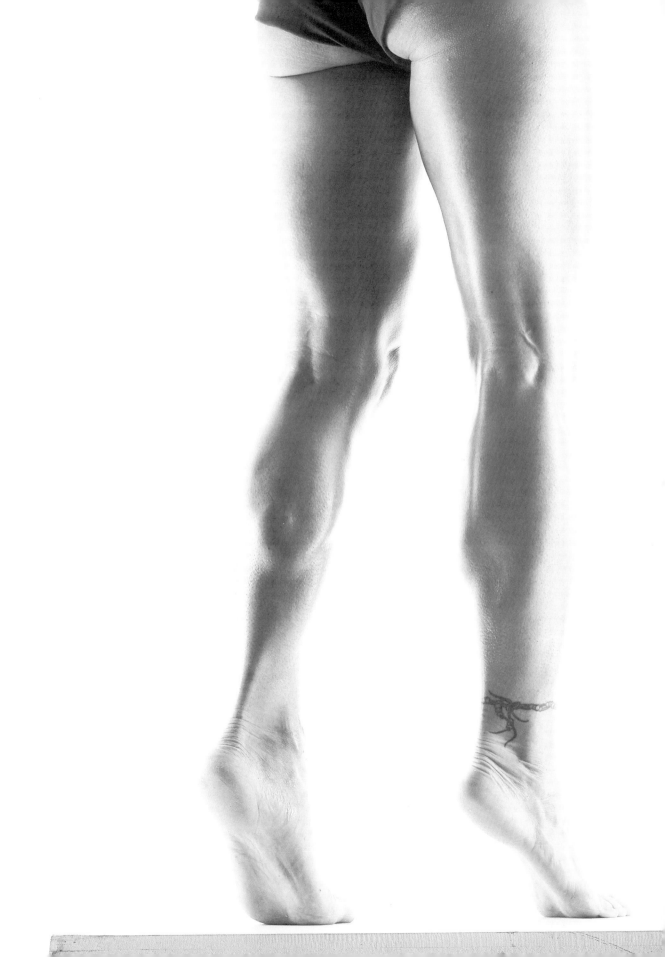

That concept certainly describes how I felt after my protein experiment was completed. Over the next four years, because of Schendel, I took more than forty graduate hours of nutrition coursework and, under his direction, I completed a postdoctoral study on nutrition and athletic performance.

BOOKS, BOOKS, BOOKS

When I finished my postdoctoral study in 1973, I immediately went to work with Arthur Jones and his Nautilus Sports/Medical Industries. Jones was highly supportive of my interest in nutrition and encouraged me to write as many articles as possible debunking high-protein powders and other food supplements. After more than two dozen articles, I had enough material—along with the research I did with Schendel—to assemble into a book.

In the early 1970s, there was not a single book available on nutrition and athletic performance by any publisher. In fact, no major publishers were the slightest bit interested. None!

After twelve months of writing letters and waiting, writing letters and waiting, I finally found a receptive, small publisher in California: the Athletic Press. They published my first book, *Nutrition and Athletic Per-*

formance, in 1976. And you know what? After all these years, this book is still in print. With absolutely no revisions or updates, it's been through dozens and dozens of printings. *Nutrition and Athletic Performance* set the stage for many other nutrition-fitness books to be published throughout the 1980s and 1990s.

Recognizing the interest, I followed up with several other books for different publishers. All of them hammered the use of supplements and health foods. Protein supplements and meal-replacement powders were deemed "unnecessary."

EDUCATED GUIDELINES

Over the past twenty years I've continued to test new meal-replacement products and food supplements. Some have been a boon, others have been a bust. Here's what I've learned.

Protein supplements. According to the Food and Nutrition Board's Recommended Dietary Allowances, adults require 0.8 grams of protein per kilogram of body weight per day. That translates into 0.36 grams per pound of body weight. If you weigh 200 pounds, for example, you need 72 grams of protein each day. In spite of some research that shows that bodybuilders require up to twice as much protein as normal people, I'm not convinced—especially since I have some personal data that show otherwise. Research reveals that protein is not a nutrient that athletes and fitness-minded people are remotely close to being deficient in. Don't waste your money on protein supplements.

Meal replacements. The technology behind meal-replacement products is far superior to what it was twenty years ago. Today, there are numerous engineered foods that are nutritious and tasty. So, yes, there's a place for meal replacements for busy people who want convenience and speed when it comes to their food. Those that I have tested, used successfully, and recommend are:

• Go Energy Shake, available from www.Go-energy-recovery.com

• Classic GROW!, available from www.BiotestEdge.com

• Ultramet, available from www.Champion-Nutrition.com

Two others that I have examined, tried, and approve of are Myoplex from EAS and MET-Rx Drink Mix. (*Note:* All five of these meal replacements are fairly high in protein and are a more appropriate source of quality protein than the vast majority of super-high-protein powders.)

Vitamin and mineral pills. I recommend that people who are trying to lose fat by reducing their calories take a multivitamin with minerals each day. This pill should:

• Provide all the RDAs in amounts smaller than or equal to the guidelines. (*Note:* The guidelines apply to eleven vitamins and seven minerals. To find their recommended safe levels, visit the Web site of the National Institute of Health's Office of Disease Prevention at http://odp.od.nih.gov and click on the link for the Office of Dietary Supplements.)

• Not supply more than the RDA of any vitamin or mineral. Remember, you get nutrients from foods, too. Plus, high-potency formulas and claims can be misleading and even dangerous.

• Not furnish substances, such as inositol and choline, which aren't needed in human nutrition. They are sometimes included in vitamin pills, as they are claimed to counter the aging process.

• Not be expensive. Local or store brands are probably just as good as nationally advertised supplements.

Ergogenic aids. Many different substances and products are marketed as performance enhancing. Remember earlier when I mentioned that large gray area between a food and a drug? Well, the regulation of ergogenic aids falls into this category where just about anything goes—at least until the market or government agrees upon how and whether to limit the claims that can be made. There are thousands of these types of products. Some of the most popular, none of which has any magical qualities, are as follows: bee pollen, branched-chain amino acids, brewer's yeast, carnitine, chromium picolinate, coenzyme Q_{10}, ginseng, herbal steroids, honey, kelp, lecithin, royal jelly, and spirulina.

Don't be bamboozled into believing that any of these products will make you bigger, leaner, faster, or stronger—at least, not any more than ordinary foods that contain the same essential nutrients. Once again, save your money.

TRAIN SMARTER: USE YOUR MIND

The search for a single food, nutrient, pill, or supplement that will safely and effectively enhance the body will continue as long as people are motivated toward excellence. When athletic performance does improve after the use of a certain product, it's usually the result of the placebo effect—the power of the mind over the body. Many people fail to recognize this power, and instead give credit to a pill or supplement.

"If you're ready to believe," an old proverb notes, "you're easy to deceive." Unfortunately, there are millions of fitness-minded people throughout the world who are being deceived. The overwhelming majority of body-enhancing food supplements are frauds. In the long run, wishful thinking is not a substitute for appropriate genetics, hard training, adequate diet, sound sleep, and mental preparedness. Don't, however, underestimate the power of your mind.

There's no reason why you can't harness the power of your own mind by believing in the science of good nutrition and sound training. Imagine yourself as you want to be and progress in a stair-step fashion toward that goal.

You don't have to buy into supplement magic to produce the results you want. You already possess plenty of magic: *your mind.*

16

SUPERHYDRATION:

A SUPERCHARGED PRACTICE

SUPERHYDRATION—YOU WON'T FIND that word in any dictionary.

I coined *superhydration* in 1988 to mean the almost continuous sipping of 1 gallon or more of ice-cold water a day, primarily to facilitate the fat-loss process.

THE ORIGINS OF SUPERHYDRATION

I didn't invent the concept of drinking large amounts of cold water, but I was the first to popularize it by connecting it to my fat-loss courses. Also, I was probably the first author to provide specific directions on why, how, and when to consume the fluid.

I did have a lot of help, however. Dr. Harold Schendel stressed the value of drinking lots of water in losing fat. Brenda Hutchins, who worked with me on many recipes in my early fat-loss studies, also made major contributions. Connie May, who trained many research subjects at the Nautilus headquarters in Dallas, had several great ideas about drinking water. And so did Terry Duschinski, the owner of a personal training center in DeLand, Florida.

Superhydration began to formalize in 1985 as I supervised three large groups of subjects through the Nautilus diet program at Joe Cirulli's fitness center in Gainesville. I instructed the groups to drink 64 ounces of water a day. Back then, I recommended that the water could be consumed at any temperature because I was unaware of the added effect of drinking it ice-cold. This research was published in *The Nautilus Diet*.

When Nautilus Sports/Medical Industries relocated their headquarters to Dallas in 1987, I continued to research and refine these ideas. These findings were published in three books: *The Six-Week Fat-to-Muscle Makeover*, *32 Days to a 32-Inch Waist*, and *Hot Hips and Fabulous Thighs*. By then I had increased my recommendation to 128 ounces of water a day and I was beginning to explore the advantages of consuming cold water.

After three years in Dallas, I returned to the Gainesville Health and Fitness Center, and from 1990 through 1997 I wrote four more books: *Two Weeks to a Tighter Tummy*, *Living Longer Stronger*, *Body Defining*, and *A Flat Stomach ASAP*. While writing these programs I proved that drinking chilled water was a significant boon to the fat-loss process. I actually had some of my subjects drink up to 2 gallons of water per day. Interestingly, the individuals who consistently drank the most cold water tended to lose the most fat.

Since the late 1980s, 551 women and 279 men have completed one of my programs that included superhydration. Not one of these participants ever suffered a medical problem as a result of drinking 1 gallon (128 ounces) of ice-cold water each day.

The reason I mention this is because superhydration has been criticized by some as problematic or dangerous. "People can't drink that much water without getting sick," noted a medical adviser who vetoed a review of one of my books from being published in a large newspaper.

They not only can drink that much water, I've discovered, *but they thrive on it.*

Let's take a closer look at why your body thrives on water.

WATER AND THE HUMAN BODY

The human body is composed of from 50 to 65 percent water. But not all body parts have the same water percentage. Your blood, for example, is 90 percent water, your brain is 85 percent, your muscle is 72 percent, your skin is 71 percent, your bone is 30 percent, and your fat is 15 percent.

As your body experiences dehydration, you feel it first in those parts that contain the most water. For example, you lose your mental alertness and suffer from overall muscular weakness. The last component that dehydration affects is your fat. That's why excessive sweating makes almost no dent in reducing your body-fat percentage.

Men have more water in their bodies than women, primarily because men have more muscle mass and less fat. A lean man of 180 pounds may have 14 gallons of water in his body. A gallon of water weighs approximately 8 pounds, so simple multiplication reveals that 112 pounds of this man's body is water.

You may not think of water as food, but it's the most critical nutrient in your daily life. You can live only a few days without it. Every process in your body requires water. For instance, it:

• Acts as a solvent for vitamins, minerals, amino acids, and glucose

• Carries nutrients throughout the body

• Makes food digestion possible

• Lubricates the joints

• Serves as a shock absorber inside the eyes and spinal cord

• Maintains body temperature

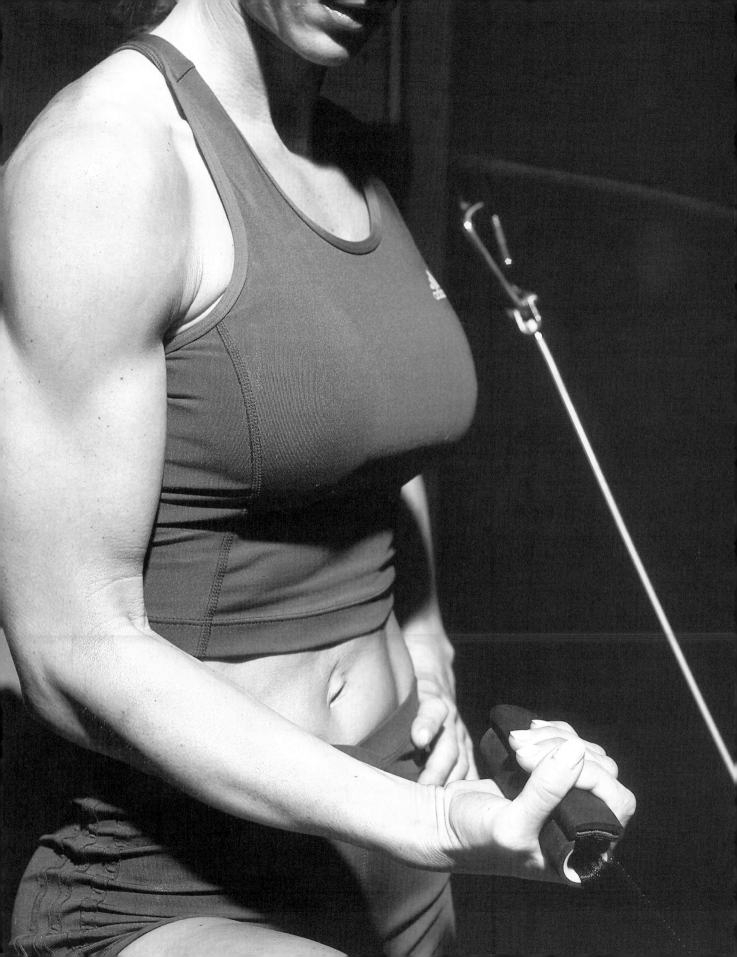

- Rids the body of waste products through the urine

- Eliminates heat through the skin, lungs, and urine

- Keeps the skin supple

- Assists muscular contraction

PARTIAL DEHYDRATION

Water contributes to so many functions that most people take it for granted. At the end of a long workday, maybe you have a headache. Plus your eyes are irritated, your back hurts, and your entire body has a dull numbness. You blame it on stress and lack of sleep.

Maybe you're right. More likely, you're simply suffering from partial dehydration.

Perhaps you had several cups of coffee for breakfast, a high-fat lunch with more coffee or maybe an alcoholic drink or two, and spent the rest of your time breathing air-conditioned or heated air at work—all of which has left your body dry and parched. Unless you've been drinking water throughout the day, dehydration is your problem.

If you are attuned and sensitive enough to your body's signals, you should be able to recognize some of the early warnings of dehydration:

- Dizziness

- Headache

- Fatigue

- Thirst

- Flushed skin

- Blurred vision

- Muscle weakness

These warning signs merit your attention. Unfortunately, most people never realize that they spend most days in a state of partial dehydration.

Although thirst is an important warning sign, many people seem to be desensitized to the signal. Some people, especially adults over forty, may actually have a decreased sensation of thirst. A good rule of thumb: Hydrate *before* you get thirsty.

WATER AND FAT LOSS

Drinking large amounts of water facilitates the fat-loss process in a number of ways.

Aids kidney and liver function. Your kidneys require abundant water to function properly. If your kidneys do not get enough water, your liver takes over and assumes some of the functions of the kidneys. This diverts your liver from its primary duty, which is to metabolize stored fat into usable energy.

If your liver is preoccupied with performing the chores of your water-depleted kidneys, it doesn't efficiently convert stored materials into usable energy. Thus, your fat loss stops, or at least plateaus. Superhydration accelerates the metabolism of fat.

Controls appetite. Lots of water flowing over your tongue keeps your taste buds cleansed of flavors that might otherwise trigger a craving. Furthermore, water keeps your stomach feeling full between meals, which can help take the edge off your appetite.

Increases urine production. Remember, as much as 85 percent of your daily heat loss emerges from your skin. Heat equals calories equals fat. That's right: Most of your fat is lost through your skin in the form of heat. The remaining 15 percent of heat loss is divided between the warm air coming from your lungs and warm fluid being passed out through urination.

Superhydration can double, triple, or even quadruple your urine production. As a result, you'll be able to eliminate more heat, calories, and fat. Get used to going to the bathroom more frequently than normal.

Burns calories. Have you ever wished for a food that supplies negative calories? Let's say such a

DON'T FORGET TO WATER YOUR CHICKENS AND YOUR FOOTBALL FIELD

Did you know that chickens need water to an even greater degree than humans? Well, at least those chickens do that lay eggs, according to Roger Lycke, an animal husbandry expert from Ocala, Florida.

Deny a laying hen water for twenty-four hours and that chicken's egg production will drop 40 percent. Stretch that out for forty-eight hours and no matter how well you hydrate the hen afterward, you'll never get another egg. Never!

Football fields need water too—and lots of it. In 2001, according to the *Orlando Sentinel*, the home fields of the Florida Gators in Gainesville and Florida State Seminoles in Tallahassee stayed green due to irrigation systems that used 9 million gallons of water. That's an average of 12,328.75 gallons of water per day for each field. A typical backyard swimming pool holds about 15,000 gallons—so, each day, a football field needs to drink almost a swimming pool of water. That's some kind of superhydration!

food exists and it contains minus 100 calories per serving. Anytime you feel like a piece of chocolate cake or a donut, all you have to do is eat two servings of the negative-calorie food. Presto—plus 200 calories and minus 200 calories yields zero calories. While no negative-calorie food exists, ice-cold water has a similar effect.

When you drink water chilled to about 40°F, your body has to use energy to heat it to your core body temperature of 98.6°. It takes almost 1 calorie to warm each ounce of cold water to body temperature. Thus, an 8-ounce glass of cold water burns approximately 8 calories—7.69 to be exact. Drink a gallon during the day and you've burned 123 calories, which is significant. *There's real calorie-burning power in cold water.*

Stops constipation. When deprived of water, your system pulls fluid from your lower intestines and bowel, creating hard, dry stools. One of the big roles of water is to flush waste from your body. This is especially important while metabolizing fat because waste tends to accumulate quickly during this process. Superhydration tends to make people more regular and consistent with their bowel movements, which is helpful to overall fat loss.

GUIDELINES FOR DRINKING WATER

How do you drink a gallon of ice-cold water a day? Although it may sound difficult, in fact, it presents only a few minor problems—such as how, when, and where. Each of these problems can be solved with some intelligent planning.

How. One secret is to not *drink* the water, but to *sip* it. Get yourself one of those 32-ounce plastic bottles, the kind that has a long straw in the top. I've found that most people consume water more easily with a straw than out of a glass. Also, while you're checking out various bottles, select one that is insulated. The insulation will keep your water colder for a longer time.

When. Drink water throughout the day. Try to consume 50 percent before noon and the rest before 6:00 P.M. Drinking most of the water early eliminates the need to get out of bed during the night to visit the bathroom.

Where. Sip water everywhere you go during the day and plan ahead. Once again, all you need is a 32-ounce, insulated plastic bottle. Really motivated people invest in a 2-gallon thermos jug. First thing in the morning, they prepare it with ice and water, fill their insulated bottle, and start sipping. As soon as the bottle is empty, they refill it from the thermos jug. When they leave home each day, they carry both the thermos jug and the smaller bottle with them. That way they always have access to their chilled water. When they return home that night, they wash the jug and the bottle and prepare for the next morning.

A great way to keep count of the bottles and ounces is to place rubber bands around the middle of the bottle equal to the number of bottles of water you are supposed to drink. Each time you finish 32 ounces, take off a rubber band. Remove four rubber bands, and you're done.

Additives. There is a difference between plain water and beverages that contain mostly water. Soft drinks, coffee, tea, beer, and fruit juices contain sugar, flavors, caffeine, and alcohol. Sugar and alcohol add calories. Caffeine stimulates the adrenal glands and acts as a diuretic. Rather than superhydrating the system, caffeine-containing beverages dehydrate the body. You should keep such beverages to a minimum. The only recommended flavoring for water is a twist of lemon or lime.

Tap water or bottled water? The United States has one of the safest water supplies in the world.

Chances are high that your community's tap water is fine for drinking. Furthermore, research shows that bottled water is not always higher quality than tap water. The decision to consume bottled water or not is usually one of taste.

If you dislike the taste of your tap water, then drink your favorite bottled water. Just be sure to check the label carefully for unwanted additives. You can also purchase one of the many home water-purifying filters that are on the market. If you have no problems with your city's water supply, then save your money and drink it.

TOO MUCH WATER

It's possible to drink too much water, but it's highly unlikely that you would ever do so. In the medical literature, drinking too much water leads to a condition know as hyponatremia. Hyponatremia most often occurs in athletes involved in triathlons and ultra-marathons. A few of these athletes consume many gallons of water during these unusually long competitions and don't or can't stop to urinate. Thus, they impede their normal fluid-mineral balance and actually become intoxicated with too much water. Such a condition, however, is rare.

I've never observed anything close to intoxication happening with any of my participants, and some of them consume 2 gallons of water daily. Of course, they also have no trouble urinating frequently.

Note: Anyone with a kidney disorder or anyone who takes diuretics should consult a physician before making modifications to his or her water consumption.

GIVE SUPERHYDRATION A TRY

If you have more than 5 pounds of fat to lose, then I'd suggest that you begin superhydration by following the plan in chapter 19. If you have only a few pounds of fat to lose, if you are already in lean condition, or if you just want to give superhydration an informal trial, then here are some guidelines.

• Purchase a 32-ounce, insulated plastic bottle to sip your water from.

• Start by sipping 1 gallon of water a day. Do not drink more during this informal trial period.

• Drink most of the water before 6:00 P.M.

• Keep the water ice-cold. Remember, each ounce of 40-degree water requires approximately 1 calorie to warm it to your core body temperature of 98.6 degrees.

• Apply the above recommendations for at least fourteen days.

THE CIRCLE OF WATER

Three million years ago, Mars must have been overflowing with oceans, seas, and rivers. Over the course of time, it lost its water, probably due to a shift in its axis of rotation. This ancient story is carved in the planet's surface with the marks made by powerful flows of water.

Water on Earth, in contrast, involves a marvel of equilibrium. The distance between the sun and Earth is almost perfect, so ground temperatures allow water to remain in a gaseous or solid state, thus preventing large-scale flooding. Without the atmospheric blanket that enshrouds and safeguards Earth, the water cycle would never have been released and the adventures of life, as we know them, would never have evolved.

The most extraordinary fact is that the water that is so present and so necessary in our lives, the water that permeates each one of our cells—this same water was there in Earth's early stages.

The circle of water: It endures without end in its three states: gas, liquid, and solid.

WHAT TO EXPECT

Expect to feel more energetic, less fatigued, smoother skinned, and more satiated by the end of the first week. Anticipate being a little leaner by the end of the second week.

If you keep the superhydration routine intact for a full month, you just may get hooked for a long time.

During this brief process, you'll come to understand that some of what you've been calling *hunger* was really an inner cry for more water. Listen closely to your body. It will reward you when it gets what it needs.

A FINAL TOAST

Superhydration has worked for thousands of people. It will work for you by improving your well-being—both on the inside and on the outside of your body. It will definitely help you lose fat and live leaner longer.

Decide today to make superhydration a salient aspect of your daily lifestyle.

Let's drink to it.

WATER: on the rocks . . . straight up . . . and with a straw.

Make it a double!

17
SLEEP:
A WAKE-UP CALL

AFTER TRAINING THOUSANDS OF OUT-OF-SHAPE people over the past twenty years, I have an observation: Participants who sleep more than eight hours per night, as compared to trainees who sleep less than eight hours, get better fat-loss results.

Too little sleep, evidently, sends a signal to your brain that your body is under stress. As a result, it shuts down—or at least limits—your system's ability to lose fat and build muscle. On the other hand, extra sleep tells your brain that everything is fine and dandy, and—presto—your system can efficiently do as directed!

To illustrate this, I want to tell you about a couple who went through one of my fat-loss programs several years ago in Gainesville.

A GAINESVILLE COUPLE

Paige and Jeff Arnold had been married for two years when I met them at an introductory meeting for my fat-loss program. They had both allowed their bodies to become fat and flabby. At that time, Paige was twenty-nine years old and weighed 150¾ pounds at a height of 5 feet 8 inches. Jeff was twenty-seven, stood 6 feet 1 inch, and weighed 219¼ pounds. Both needed to lose fat from their bodies. They signed up and began my supervised six-week program.

I weigh all my subjects before each workout. Jeff's numbers over the first two weeks were 219, 215, 211, 208, and 204. In 14 days, Jeff lost 15 pounds.

Paige's numbers, however, were quite different. Even though Paige and Jeff were both following the basic eating and exercising plan, her numbers were 150, 153, 152, 150, and 150. In two weeks, Paige did not lose a single pound. You can imagine how she felt—disgusted and depressed.

I talked with both of them. It didn't take me long to realize that Paige was not getting enough sleep. She worked at a radio station in Gainesville and had to get up most mornings at 4:00 A.M. Most nights she was lucky to sleep for five hours.

Jeff, however, had no problem with sleep. Most nights he never even felt Paige ease out of bed at 4:00 A.M. and couldn't remember the radio playing loud music as Paige dressed. Nine hours per night was the norm for Jeff.

Anyway, after explaining to Paige the importance of getting additional rest, she rearranged her schedule and got on track for more sleep. She rebounded by losing 7 pounds over the next two weeks and another 7½ pounds over the last two weeks of the program—14½ pounds of fat in four weeks. Jeff continued his steady reduction and at the end of six weeks had lost 33½ pounds of fat.

Paige and Jeff continued with my program for another six weeks. After twelve weeks, Paige removed 25¾ pounds of fat and Jeff 54¼ pounds. Both added more than 5 pounds of muscle to their physiques.

"Getting abundant sleep made the difference for me," Paige noted. "Initially, my fat loss seemed to be on hold. The extra sleep was the catalyst I needed to get the results I wanted."

HOW MUCH SLEEP IS ENOUGH?

Years ago researchers focused on sleep only as a brain phenomenon, ignoring its effects on other parts of the body. Now, they recognize that sleep regulates body temperature, replenishes the immune system, and yields hormones that facilitate fat loss and muscle building. To better understand, let's explore some of the latest facts about sleep.

An infant sleeps fourteen hours a day; a teenager averages nine and a half hours; and people over seventy-five years old manage only six hours. We sleep less as we age. The latest figures from the National Sleep Foundation show that the average adult in the United States gets 6 hours and 57 minutes of sleep per night during the workweek and 7 hours and 31 minutes during weekends. This is not enough sleep, according to the NSF, which recommends that adults get eight hours of sleep each night.

What happens when you get too little sleep? Lack of sleep for even a few nights, notes Dr. Eve Van Cauter, a University of Chicago sleep researcher, increases brain levels of cortisol, a potentially dangerous stress hormone. High levels of cortisol contribute to a number of problems, including weakening of the immune system, brain cell reduction, depression, irritability, lack of energy, and the storage of fat.

New studies indicate that the length of sleep is not what causes you to feel refreshed as much as the number of sleep cycles you complete. One sleep cycle lasts an average of 90 minutes, which is typically divided into 65 minutes of normal sleep, 20 minutes of rapid eye movement (REM) sleep (in which you dream), and another 5 minutes of normal sleep. During the night, the REM sleep phase tends to be shorter during earlier cycles and longer during later ones. Still, each cycle tends to remain constant at about 90 minutes.

Interestingly, a person who sleeps only four cycles, or six hours, will feel more rested than someone who has slept for eight or ten hours but has not finished any one sleep cycle because of restlessness or being awakened.

You are probably getting too little sleep for maximum fat loss and strength building and could profit from adding at least one more 90-minute cycle to your sleep each night. The best way to initiate this sleep pattern is to go to bed earlier rather than sleep later. Try it for a month and I bet you'll feel better as your body becomes leaner and stronger.

EXAMPLES OF EXCESSIVE STRESS

There seems to be a clear relationship between a lack of sleep and too much stress in a person's life. It seems cyclical, since getting quality sleep tends to help a person cope more effectively with stress, and dealing with stress effectively tends to allow a person to sleep better.

How does too much stress provide a major hurdle to losing fat? Some of the answer goes back to cortisol, one of your body's primary stress-related hormones.

Cortisol, released by your adrenal gland, prepares your body to take action. Production of the hormone subsides once the action is over. But if the stressful event doesn't end or continues to perturb you, then some of the hormone remains in your system.

Studies in animals and older people show long-term exposure to high levels of cortisol can damage brain cells, shrink the hippocampus (a critical region of the brain that regulates learning and memory), and, as I mentioned earlier, promote the storing of lipids in your fat cells.

Here is a listing of physical stresses that can cause your body to hold on to fat:

• *A very low-calorie diet:* Under 1,200 calories a day for men and 1,000 calories a day for women

• *Too little dietary fat:* Fewer than 30 grams a day for men and 20 grams a day for women

• *Too much strength training or other types of exercise:* Longer than 45 minutes per workout, or more frequently than three times per week

• *Too little sleep:* Less than six hours per night

• *Dehydration:* A loss of 1 percent of the body's water can cause alarm

• *Excessive heat:* High levels of environmental heat can reduce the body's efficiency

• *Accumulated problems:* Business and relationship conflicts can have negative effects

• *Sicknesses, drugs, or extreme behaviors:* Almost anything out of the ordinary can send survival signals to the body

For maximum fat loss, you want to communicate to your body that everything is well. You do this best by avoiding excessive stress and by practicing moderation in almost everything—except your strength training.

Moderately intense strength training is not very productive. Strength training that is performed slowly and smoothly for maximum repetitions is stressful—as it must be—to stimulate the fastest possible muscular growth. That's why it's important to keep your strength training brief.

But wait a minute. How does muscular growth stimulation send a positive message to your system to part with its fat? Once again, we must look to our ancestors for the answer.

STRENGTH AND SURVIVAL

One of the basic necessities of our ancestors' lives was movement. Movement depended on muscular strength. Anthropological research shows that survival depended, in part, on the ability to run fast and fight fiercely to eat and avoid being eaten. Hard, brief activity produced stronger muscles, and stronger muscles led to success at hunting and in battle. Stronger, larger muscles improved the probability of survival.

Today, when you go on a reduced-calorie diet, your body perceives stress—that something is wrong. Cortisol is released, which, if sustained long enough, will prevent you from losing fat in the most efficient manner.

To combat this situation, learn to deal with your stresses quickly and productively. Do not let your troubles linger. Be proactive. And, most important, stimulate your muscles to grow with proper strength training, then rest fully, which means getting plenty of sleep. Then, and only then, will your muscles draw calories for growth from your fat cells, which increases the effectiveness and efficiency of your ability to reduce fat.

YOU'RE SLEEPY

Listen to me carefully.

You are getting sleepy. Your eyes are feeling very heavy. Your head is beginning to nod. You can already feel the great rewards of a pleasant night of peaceful sleep.

Close this book now. Retreat to your bedroom and let your *body* do the *rest*.

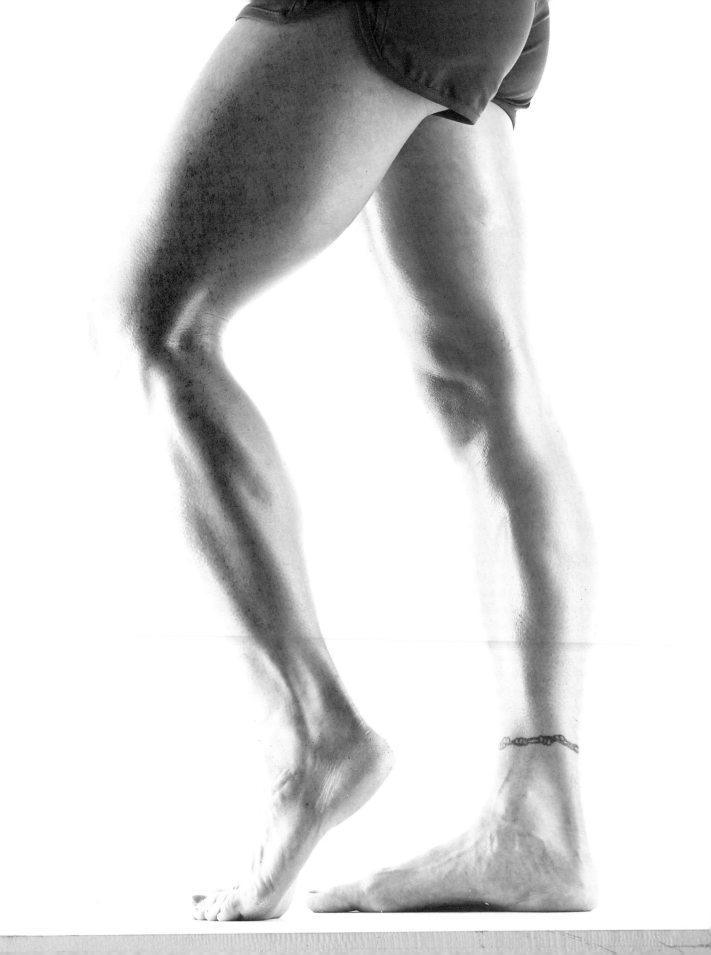

18

SYNERGY:

$$1 + 1 + 1 = 5$$

SYNERGY IS THE SIMULTANEOUS action of separate things that, together, have a greater total effect than the sum of their individual effects. In medicine, a drug that aids or cooperates with another drug is said to be a synergist. Muscles working together, as the pectorals, deltoids, and triceps do in a bench press, are described as synergistic. If synergy applied to mathematics, then 1 + 1 + 1 *could* equal 5 or even more.

There's a lot of synergy that takes place in the human body, during the processes of building muscle and losing fat. I've witnessed this in dozens of participants who have completed my six-week programs and built more muscle or lost more fat than they expected. When a person gets the exercising, eating, cooling, superhydrating, and sleeping all in the right proportions, then synergy kicks in big time.

Two people come to mind immediately. The first is Eddie Mueller, a young man who wanted to build his muscles. The second is Larry Freedman, who had a lot of fat to lose. Their stories will prove inspiring.

Note: For comparison, an average man who goes through one of my programs can expect to build 0.625 pounds of muscle a week—or 3.75 pounds of muscle in six weeks. That same man can expect to lose 3.58 pounds of fat a week—or 21.5 pounds of fat in six weeks. Keep these figures in mind as you read about Eddie and Larry.

EDDIE MUELLER: GETTING BIG

Mueller was so motivated to build muscle that during the summer of 1989 he moved from Florida to Texas. He wanted to be a part of a six-week program I was conducting at the Nautilus headquarters in Dallas.

At twenty-three years of age and a height of 5 feet 8¾ inches, Mueller weighed 172½ pounds at the start of the program. He had strength trained off and on since high school, so he was in above-average shape with his body fat at 6.9 percent. I personally trained Mueller three times per week on ten exercises, using some of the intermediate and advanced techniques described in chapters 9 and 10. None of his workouts ever lasted longer than 30 minutes.

Eating was an important aspect of his success. Since Mueller had a high metabolism, to calculate the number of calories that he should consume each day I took his body weight and multiplied it by 20. Then, to this number I added 500 calories. On average, Mueller consumed more than 4,000 calories per day in six meals. And he drank at least a gallon of water each day.

At the end of the six-week course, Mueller weighed 192 pounds. He gained 19½ pounds, or an average of 3¼ pounds per week. In the process, he added 1½ inches on his upper arms, 5 inches on his chest, and 4⅞ inches on his thighs. But not all of that 19½ pounds was muscle. Skin fold measurements revealed that his body fat increased from 6.9 to 8.8 percent. Calculations showed that 5 of the 19½ pounds were fat. Still, Mueller added 14½ pounds of muscle to his body in six weeks.

Most of Mueller's fat accumulation was around his midsection. As with many athletes who want to gain weight, I've found that it's easier to build muscle by adding calories as opposed to keeping calories at a moderate level. After the initial weight gain, then, they can lose the unwanted fat. Mueller's midsection fat, in fact, was off less than two weeks after he had completed the program.

LARRY FREEDMAN: THE GRAND CHAMPION OF FAT LOSS

Freedman was the most motivated of a group of fifteen people who went through my six-week fat-loss course in April of 1993 at the Gainesville Health and Fitness Center. At 5 feet 11 inches he weighed 306 pounds and his waist measured 52⅝ inches. He was twenty-nine years old at that time.

As far as the group was concerned, Freedman had the ideal combination of seriousness and humor. He was both the group's father confessor and their head cheerleader. And Freedman used group dynamics to his advantage. He wasn't about to get caught cheating on any of the exercising or eating. The results starting showing almost immediately on Freedman's body.

After six weeks, Freedman had lost 52¾ pounds of fat, for an average per week rate of 8.79 pounds, and an average daily rate of 1.26 pounds. In my forty years of working with overfat people, I've never had anyone lose 50 or more pounds in six weeks. Freedman is my grand champion of fat loss.

And that was just the start. Freedman continued the program for another four months. At the end of six months, Freedman had dropped 116½ pounds of fat and built 5½ pounds of muscle. He lost 15½ inches off his waist, 11⅛ inches off his hips, and 15⅜ inches off his thighs. His body weight went from 306 to 195 pounds and his body fat shrunk from 45 percent to 10.9 percent.

MUSCULAR SYNERGY

Both Mueller and Freedman became experts at synergy. In their groups, each led by being an example to others. Neither one cheated on his diet and their strength-training commitment grew as they progressed, reached, and exceeded their goals.

Remember, besides making you look, feel, and perform better, strength training speeds up your metabolism. Add a pound of muscle to your body through Bowflex exercise, and your metabolism increases by approximately 37.5 calories per day. The average man who adds 3.75 pounds of muscle to his body during my program will burn 140.6 more calories per day. Over twenty-five days that's 1 pound of body fat.

Recall also that fatty tissue influences metabolism: Fat needs only 2 calories per pound a day to keep it functioning while muscle demands 37.5 calories.

It should be clear by now that losing fat without building muscle is not a good idea and only lowers metabolism. Adding as little as 1 pound of muscle compensates for the metabolic loss of almost 19 pounds of fat.

Build as much muscle as you can—5 or even 10 pounds—in the next six months or so. Muscles are like a compound, interest-bearing savings account. Building larger, stronger muscles is true synergy in action.

OTHER SYNERGISTIC FACTORS

Besides your exercising, eating, cooling, superhydrating, and sleeping practices, there are a few other factors that can contribute to fat loss. You should consider each one.

• Ask a friend to progress through the Bowflex program with you. You'll probably get better results if you work your program with a friend. Both you and your friend should be serious about making a commitment. That commitment means you'll be exercising together three times per week, pushing each other through those difficult repetitions, talking on the phone often, perhaps eating together, and sharing problems.

• Avoid strenuous activity or other exercise on the days you do not train on Bowflex. Too much activity can be more harmful than too little activity, especially while following a low-calorie diet. If you are trying to lose fat and build muscle at the same time, keep activity outside the program to a minimum. Certainly, you should continue with your normal work and household responsibilities, but avoid rigorous activities such as running, basketball, skiing, aerobic classes, and swimming. Light recreational games not carried to extremes are probably fine, but if in doubt don't do them. Once you reach your fat-loss goal, you can get involved in other strenuous sports and fitness endeavors if you wish.

• Walk moderately after your evening meal. If you walk at a leisurely pace for 30 minutes with food and cold water in your belly, you'll significantly speed up your body's ability to release heat and burn calories. Begin your walks within 15 minutes of finishing your meal. Your goal is to cover 1½ to 2 miles in 30 minutes. Wear well-constructed and comfortable walking or running shoes. Walk outdoors, if possible, on level ground. Or you may substitute a bicycle ride for the walk. If the weather is a problem, walk indoors or use a stationary bicycle or a treadmill.

• Incorporate good posture. Proper posture burns more calories than poor posture. Correct posture automatically forces you to tighten your midsection muscles. The best posture resembles a marionette with a string attached to the top of the head. Imagine being gently tugged upward by the string. This applies well to sitting, standing, and walking. Good posture emphasizes leanness.

• Watch only essential television programs. TV exposes you to advertisements that know how to prompt you to buy and to eat. Such advertising has its fingers on all our impulse buttons. Make it a rule never to eat while watching TV. Instead of TV, get outside for a walk, retire to bed earlier, or read a book—all these will help you break the evening TV habit.

• Be proactive. Refocus your eating around conscious choices based on tried-and-proven guidelines, as opposed to making reactive choices, which flow from physical and social environments. Learn to simply say NO to certain foods and temptations, and YES to things that are beneficial to your strength and leanness.

BETTER RESULTS FASTER

Synergy allows you to get better results faster. Be proactive right now, and choose to apply the synergistic factors throughout your Bowflex program.

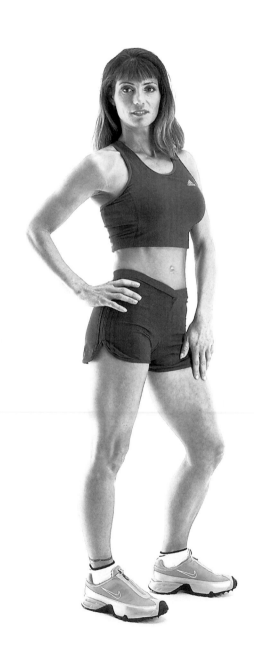

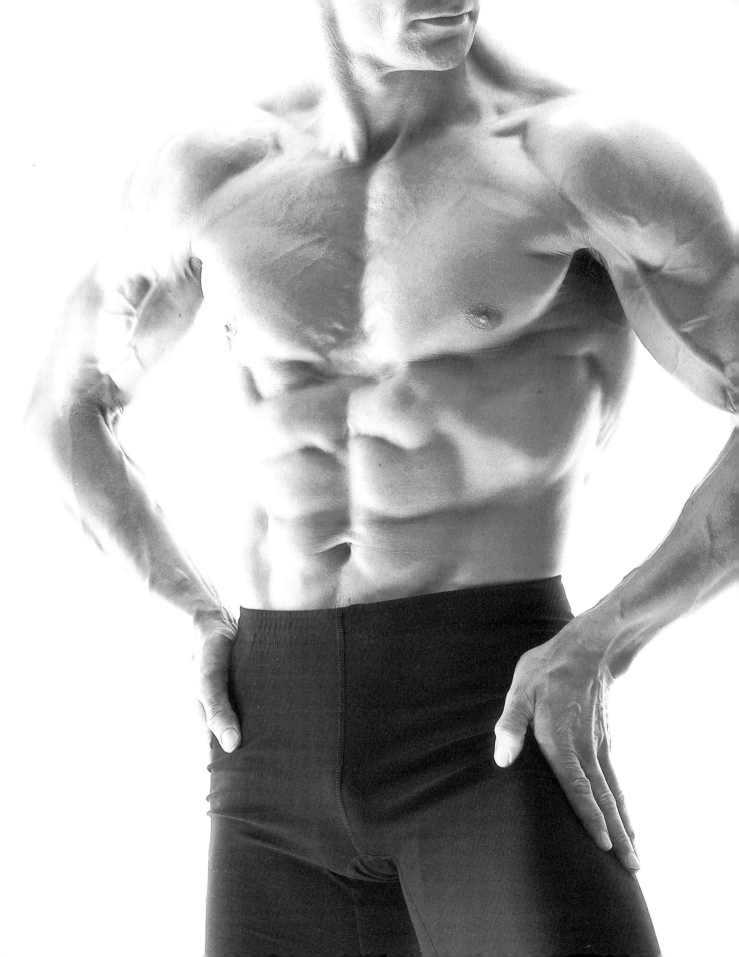

19

PREPARATION:

WHAT TO DO FIRST

EACH OF THE NEXT FOUR chapters involves a reduced-calorie eating plan. Such a plan requires preparation, especially if you're interested in getting the best possible results. Before beginning any program, however, please do the following.

CHECK WITH YOUR PHYSICIAN

Should you call your doctor and schedule a routine physical examination? Actually, because of the prevalence of obesity in this country, most Americans should get their doctor's permission to *not* exercise and to *not* diet. There is certainly more risk involved in pursuing a sedentary, high-calorie lifestyle. Nevertheless, I recommend that you check with your physician and take this book along with you for easy referral.

There are a few groups of people who should not try a reduced-calorie eating plan: children and teenagers; pregnant women; women who are breast-feeding; men and women with certain types of heart, liver, or kidney disease; diabetics; and those suffering from some types of arthritis and cancer. Some people should follow a certain program only with their physician's specific guidance. Consult your health care professional beforehand and play it safe.

RECORD YOUR HEIGHT AND WEIGHT

Remove your clothing and shoes and record your height to the nearest quarter inch and your weight to the nearest quarter pound. Be sure to use the same scale each time you record your weight. For the most accurate recordings, weigh yourself nude in the morning.

DO CIRCUMFERENCE MEASUREMENTS

These measurements are meaningful because they let you know what is happening in specific areas of your body. Use a flexible tape to measure the following:

• Upper arms—hanging and relaxed, midway between the shoulder and elbow.

• Two inches above navel—belly relaxed.

• At navel level—belly relaxed.

• Two inches below navel—belly relaxed.

• Hips—with feet together and buttocks relaxed.

• Upper thighs—just below the buttocks crease with legs apart and weight distributed equally on both feet.

Serious Safety for a Father of Four

James M. Kelley, Jr., thirty-four, is a computer technologist in Mount Juliet, Tennessee. He's married and has four small children.

"Because of our four kids, I take exercising at home very seriously," James noted. "I love the fact that the Bowflex machine is safe. With the Power Rods I don't have to worry about heavy weight plates or dumbbells being left out for my kids' play. Of course, they need to stand clear of the Power Rods when they're in use, but still they're very safe compared to standard free weights."

James purchased a Power Pro XTL on January 26, 2001. He applied the circuit training routine three times per week because he wanted to lose about 30 pounds from his 5-foot, 7-inch frame and attain more muscle definition. He didn't follow the Body-Leanness Plan; he simply cut back on his sweets. "It took a while," James noted, "but after seven months I started seeing some wonderful changes."

Those wonderful changes amounted to a loss of 34½ pounds of fat and 4 inches off his waist. As a result his arms, chest, midsection, and legs have more muscular size and definition.

Has anyone noticed a difference in James's physique?

"My family, friends, and coworkers have all noticed and commented on how great I look," James said. "They all ask me how I did it and I reply, 'Working out on my Bowflex.' Not only does my body look better, but I have more energy and stamina for work, family, and sports such as hiking, basketball, and tennis."

In the seven months since James lost his 34½ pounds, he hasn't gained any of them back.

"I finally decided to get rid of all my old clothes," James said proudly. "They fit too loosely, even with a cinched-up belt. I rounded them all up, dropped them off at Goodwill, and said good-bye.

"Afterward, I bought all new pants, shorts, and shirts. As I walked out of the mall, I thought to myself: *Hello world, I'm a new man!* Then, I went home, hugged my wife and kids . . . and worked out."

One more thing: It's difficult to take your own measurements accurately. You'll get truer numbers if you have someone else do them for you.

CALCULATE PERCENT BODY FAT

As I stated in chapter 12, in the hands of a trained technician, skin fold calipers can supply some valu-

Teamwork: She Lost a Little, He Lost a Lot

Joshua and Dawn Caskey were recently married and live in Cloverdale, California. Joshua, twenty-six, is an engineer and Dawn, twenty, doesn't work outside the home. A history of obesity runs in Joshua's family and he has been overweight his entire life. Dawn has always been trim, except during the past year, when she put on 20 pounds.

They ordered their Bowflex machine in June 2001. They both wanted to lose weight: Dawn a little (at 5 feet 1 inches she weighed 125 pounds) and Joshua a lot (at 6 feet 4 inches he weighed more than 350 pounds). And, perhaps most important, they decided to lose weight together, as a couple, as a team.

"We grocery-shopped together, cooked together, ate together, drank water together, and exercised together," Dawn said. "Doing so helped us keep our focus." The plan worked—and is still working.

Dawn reached her goal—eliminating 20 pounds—in the first six weeks. "I watch my weight real closely now," Dawn commented. "If my body weight goes up even a pound, from 106 to 107, I focus harder and it comes off quickly."

Joshua, on the other hand, is only halfway to reaching his goal. "I've lost 60 pounds using the Body-Leanness Plan and it took me three months to do so. I know that I need to get rid of another 60 pounds or more.

"Drinking water has been very important for me. I carry a gallon jug of water with me to work each day. Now, I sip water instead of soft drinks. And you know what? A lot of my coworkers are doing the same thing. I'm seeing more and more water jugs around the office.

"At one time, because of my body weight, I couldn't even sign up for life insurance. Now, thanks to Bowflex, I'm on the road to long-life assurance."

able numbers on fat loss and muscle gain. Unfortunately, most people don't have access to calipers. If you have access to skin fold calipers, the *Bowflex Owner's Manual and Fitness Guide*, pages 65–68, shows you how to apply them and calculate your percent body fat. You can download it by going to the Web site www.Bowflex.com. Otherwise, I recommend having it done at your local fitness center.

CONSIDER FULL-BODY PHOTOGRAPHS

There is no better way to evaluate your current physical condition, and mark progress along the way, than to have full-body photographs taken of yourself in a small, revealing bathing suit. Here are good procedures to follow:

• Keep everything the same each time you're photographed. Wear the same suit each time—a snug solid color is best—and have the person taking the picture stand in the same place, with the same setting behind you.

• Stand against an uncluttered, light-colored background.

• Have the person with the camera move away from you until he can see your entire body in the viewfinder.

• Stand relaxed for three pictures: front, right side, and back. Do not suck in your stomach.

• Interlace your fingers and place them on top of your head for all three poses, so the contours of your torso will be plainly visible. Keep your feet 8 inches apart for the front and back shots, but together for the side picture.

• Make sure the film processor prints the photographs the same size each time so that comparisons can more easily be made.

PREPARE TO SUPERHYDRATE

I've already described how drinking plenty of cold water each day is essential to the success of your program. Get yourself a 32-ounce, insulated plastic bottle with a big straw—if you don't already have one—and prepare to adhere to the following schedule:

• Week 1: Drink four 32-ounce bottles of ice water each day.

• Week 2: Drink four-and-a-half 32-ounce bottles of ice water each day.

• Week 3: Drink five 32-ounce bottles of ice water each day.

• Week 4: Drink five-and-a-half 32-ounce bottles of ice water each day.

• Week 5: Drink six 32-ounce bottles of ice water each day.

• Week 6: Drink six-and-a-half 32-ounce bottles of ice water each day.

You'll be sipping and drinking from 1 to 1⅝ gallons of water each day. Don't be alarmed if you have to make more than a dozen trips to the rest room, especially during the first week. Your body will soon adapt to the increased water consumption.

TAKE A VITAMIN/MINERAL TABLET EACH DAY

I recommend that you take one multivitamin with minerals each morning with breakfast. Make sure no nutrient listed on the label exceeds 100 percent of the Recommended Dietary Allowances. High-potency supplements are not necessary.

BUY MEASURING SPOONS, CUPS, AND A SMALL SCALE

Most people have a tendency to overestimate the size of 1 ounce of cheese, 2 ounces of chicken breast, or 4 ounces of orange juice. Such practices lead to inaccurate calorie counting and ineffective fat loss. It's important to become familiar with and correctly use measuring spoons, cups, and food scales.

I recommend buying a battery-operated digital scale instead of the less expensive, spring-loaded type. Digital scales tend to be more accurate.

GIVE ATTENTION TO OTHER SYNERGISTIC ACTIVITIES

The big three elements to align for maximum synergy are reduced-calorie eating, strength training, and superhydration. But don't forget about the other mechanisms, such as sleeping and resting, keeping cool, walking after your evening meal, cutting back on TV, and practicing good posture. They all add up to make a big difference in the degree of your fat loss, muscle building, and overall success.

GET EXCITED AND BE PATIENT

You're now well prepared to begin your specific program. Your excitement is essential, but you must also have patience. Physiological changes to your body take time. *The Bowflex Body Plan* will make a difference in your life.

Let's get started.

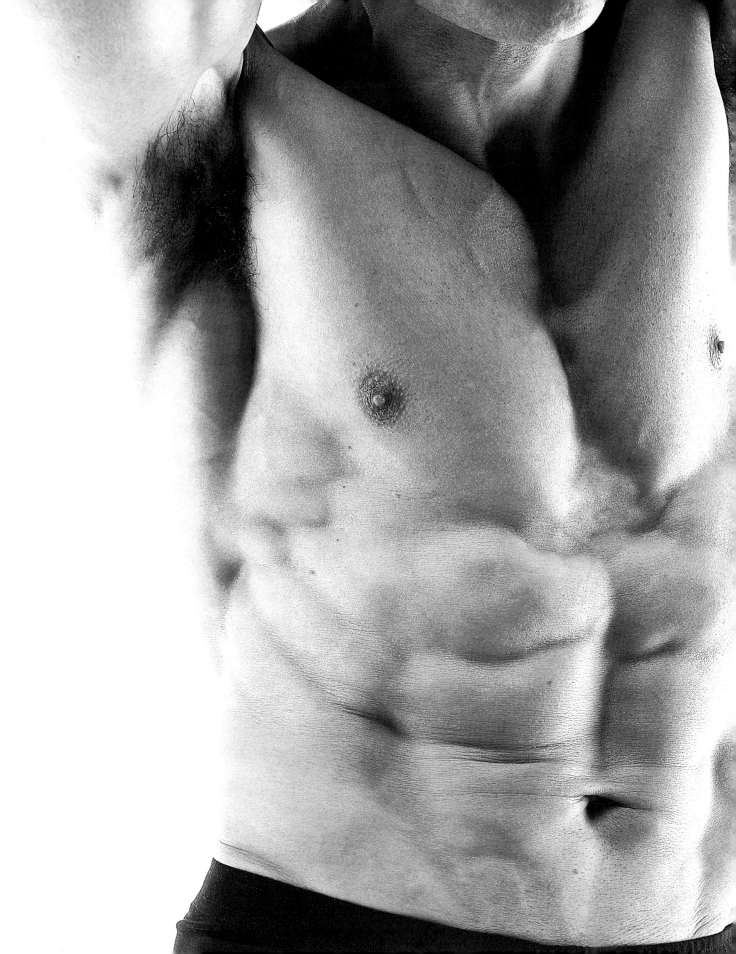

20

THE BODY-LEANNESS PLAN:

A SIX-WEEK COURSE FOR LOSING FAT

"STARTING TOMORROW," THE SMILING American announces, reaching for another piece of strawberry cheesecake, "I'm going on a diet." How many times have we heard, or repeated, that statement?

More than 165 million Americans are obese, and this problem is spreading rapidly throughout the industrialized world. More than 1.7 billion people worldwide need to lose fat.

Unfortunately, it takes no discipline to go on a diet after a big meal. That stuffed feeling and a super-tight waistband are usually all that is required. But several days later, when we're feeling deprived, it's a different matter. That's when we need all the discipline, self-control, and help we can get. Sooner or later, the mind and belly must work together to understand and apply the best that science has to offer about losing fat.

That's what the Body-Leanness Plan was designed to do: *Provide the best scientific guidelines on losing fat.* Since 1995, thousands and thousands of Bowflex owners have been through this six-week program and have achieved great results.

UNRAVELING THE CONFUSION

What I've learned from these participants reinforces what I discovered years ago. Namely:

• People are not lazy by choice. They are forced into it by the confusion and abundance of fitness information. When individuals are given simple, decisive instructions, they train intensely.

• When provided with specific menus, people will drastically alter their eating habits.

• Most people, however, will not stay with a new exercise program or diet for more than a week unless they quickly see and feel changes in their bodies.

To get the best results from the Body-Leanness Plan, you must be willing to exercise intensely on the Bowflex machine, adhere to a strict eating plan, superhydrate daily, and practice a lot of the little things that I discussed in Part III. In return, you'll see the pounds disappear from your body on a weekly basis.

Before I get into the details of the program, I want to share again the results of my first Bowflex research study, performed at the Gainesville Health and Fitness Center in 1995. I mentioned this study in chapter 1, and the results turned me into a Bowflex believer.

THE BOWFLEX
FAT-LOSS STUDY

Three men and three women from Gainesville were referred to me by previous participants in my programs. At the start of the plan, the men had an average body weight of 228.7 pounds, a height of 6 feet 1 inch, and an age of 33.3 years. The women had an average starting body weight of 161.7 pounds, height of 5 feet 7¾ inches, and age of 40 years.

For six weeks, the men consumed an average of 1,400 calories per day and the women 1,100 calories. Each participant drank 165 ounces of cold water each day and trained three times per week on a Bowflex machine. Here are the results.

Weight and fat loss. The men lost an average of 24.25 pounds; the women lost 14.23 pounds. The average body fat percentage for men was 26.43 before and 15.93 after. For women it was 27.87 before and 19.23 after—for an average fat loss of 27.95 pounds per man and 16.96 pounds per woman, or 4.66 pounds of fat per week for men and 2.83 pounds of fat per week for women.

Muscle gain and inches loss. Subtracting each subject's weight loss from his or her fat loss

showed that the men had an average muscle gain of 3.7 pounds and the women 2.73 pounds. Circumference measurements, before and after, were taken two inches above the navel, at the navel, two inches below the navel, and at the hips and thighs. Since people lose fat differently around the midsection, the largest before-and-after change from the three measurements was used as a subject's final waist measurement.

AVERAGE INCHES LOST

	Waist	Hips	Thighs
Men	5.790	1.625	3.625
Women	4.250	2.250	2.875

Photo comparison. Before and after photographs of each participant on the following pages reveal that visible changes were dramatic.

DISCUSSION OF STUDY

As I mentioned in chapter 1, the Bowflex men and women established new group records for fat loss compared to all previous participants in my programs. But why? What separated this group of three

BOYD WELSCH'S RESULTS

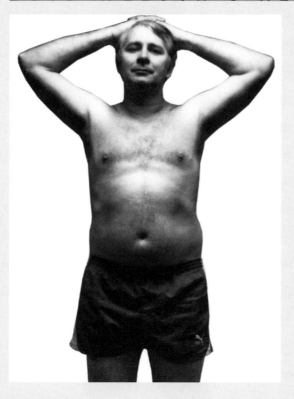 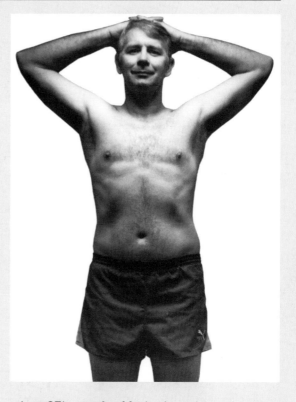

AGE: **48**
HEIGHT: **6'1"**
BEFORE WEIGHT: **232¾ POUNDS**
BEFORE WAIST SIZE: **43¼"**

- Lost **27½ pounds** of fat in six weeks
- Built **5¼ pounds** of muscle
- Trimmed **5¾"** off waist

men and three women from other groups that I worked with in the past?

The first difference that comes to mind is compliance. There was 100-percent compliance on each Bowflex workout. No one missed a single workout in

six weeks. Compliance was also excellent on the eating plan (97 percent), superhydration (88 percent), and walking after the evening meal (84 percent). Judging from these high compliance levels, they were clearly motivated. But why were they so motivated?

In my opinion, it was because they understood how overfat and out of shape they were at the start of the program. Then, the Body-Leanness Plan and Bowflex offered them practical guidelines to produce results they could see and feel quickly.

BOTTOM LINE

The Body-Leanness Plan worked because it works when people work, and these people were dedicated workers.

Can you expect similar fat-loss results to those of Boyd Welsch, who lost 27½ pounds, or Barb Welsch, who lost 16¼ pounds? Maybe you'll exceed what Nancy Young accomplished—or even Barry Ozer, who dropped almost 61 pounds in twelve weeks.

Achieving their level of success is entirely possible, but only if you have the same dedication as Boyd, Barb, Nancy, or Barry. You know your level of dedication better than anyone. From my experience, however, if you've read this far in this book, you're already well ahead of the average person on dedication and motivation.

But enough of the pep talks. If you want to benefit from the Body-Leanness Plan, then all the details follow.

THE BODY-LEANNESS ROUTINES

Here are the Bowflex routines to follow for the program:

WEEKS 1 AND 2

1. Leg Curl

2. Leg Extension

3. Bench Press

4. Standing Biceps Curl

5. Seated Shoulder Press

6. Seated Abdominal Crunch

WEEKS 3 AND 4

1. Leg Curl

2. Leg Extension

3. Lying Shoulder Pullover*

4. Seated Row*

5. Bench Press

6. Standing Biceps Curl

7. Seated Shoulder Press

8. Seated Abdominal Crunch

*New exercise

WEEKS 5 AND 6

1. Leg Curl

2. Leg Extension

BARB WELSCH'S RESULTS

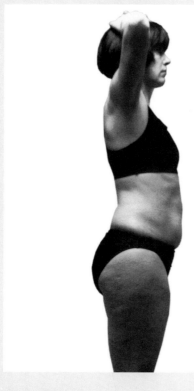 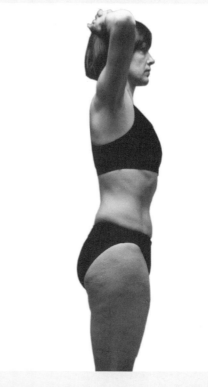

AGE: **44**

HEIGHT: **5'9"**

BEFORE WEIGHT: **154¾ POUNDS**

BEFORE WAIST SIZE: **34⅛"**

- Lost **16¼ pounds** of fat in six weeks
- Built **2½ pounds** of muscle
- Trimmed **5¾"** off waist
- Dropped **3¼"** off thighs

3. Leg Press*

4. Seated Calf Raise*

5. Lying Shoulder Pullover

6. Seated Row

7. Bench Press

8. Standing Biceps Curl

9. Seated Shoulder Press

10. Seated Abdominal Crunch

*New exercise

NANCY YOUNG'S RESULTS

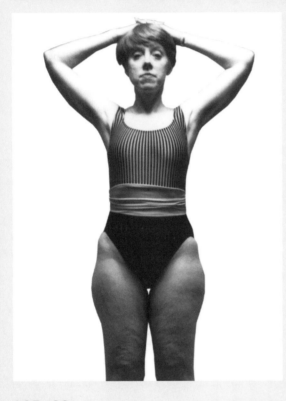 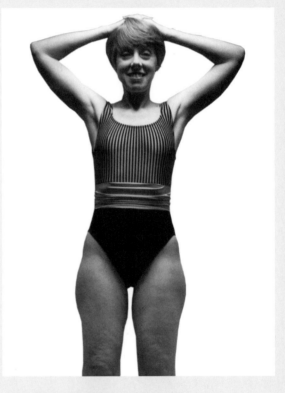

AGE: **39**
HEIGHT: **5'5"**
BEFORE WEIGHT: **141¼ POUNDS**
BEFORE WAIST SIZE: **32⅛"**

- Lost **16¼ pounds** of fat in six weeks
- Built **1¾ pounds** of muscle
- Trimmed **3⅝"** off waist
- Eliminated **3½"** off hips
- Dropped **3¾"** off thighs

You'll notice that I add two new exercises after each two-week segment. As you progress, try to reduce the time you spend going from one exercise to the next. For example, during weeks 1 and 2, allow 60 seconds between exercises. During weeks 3 and 4, reduce the time to 45 seconds. And once you're into weeks 5 and 6, limit your time between exercises to 30 seconds.

Perform one set of each exercise for 8 to 12 repetitions. Keep all repetitions smooth and slow, approximately 3 seconds on the positive and 3 seconds on the negative phase. Anytime you can do 12 or more repetitions on any exercise, add 10 pounds of Power Rods (5 pounds on each side) on your next workout. Train three nonconsecutive days per week—or eighteen times in six weeks.

THE BODY-LEANNESS SUPERHYDRATION SCHEDULE

You'll be following the week-by-week superhydration schedule on page 177 for the next six weeks. You also may want to review chapter 16 to get fired up on the benefits of this practice.

THE BODY-LEANNESS EATING PLAN

The menus in the eating plan are designed for maximum fat-loss and nutritional value. For best results, follow them exactly.

Every attempt has been made to keep current the brand names and calorie counts listed in the menus. But products are sometimes changed or discontinued. If a menu item is not available in your area, substitute a similar product.

Become an informed label reader at your supermarket as you shop. Ask questions about any products you don't understand. Supermarket managers are usually helpful. Many companies now have Web sites that provide detailed nutritional facts about their products.

Each day you will select foods from the menu for breakfast and lunch. I've found that most people can consume the same basic breakfast and the same basic lunch for months with little or no modification. Variety during your evening meal, however, makes eating interesting and enjoyable. The eating plan also includes a midafternoon and a late-night snack to keep your energy high and your hunger low.

Begin week 1 on Monday and continue through Sunday. Week 2 is a repeat of week 1. Calories for each food are noted in parentheses. A shopping list follows at the end.

The eating plan for the next six weeks descends as follows:

Weeks 1 and 2:

Men: 1,500 calories per day

Women: 1,200 calories per day

BARRY OZER'S RESULTS

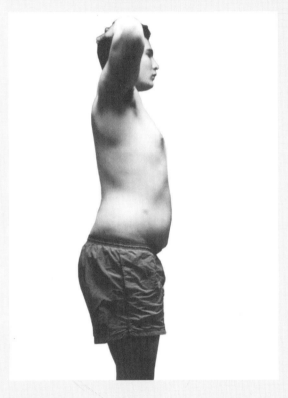 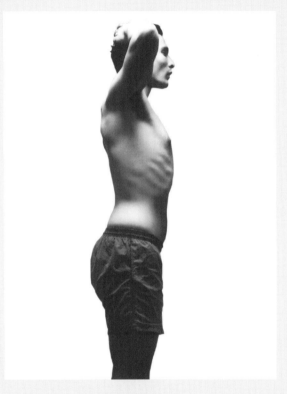

AGE: **25**

HEIGHT: **6'2"**

BEFORE WEIGHT: **239¼ POUNDS**

BEFORE WAIST SIZE: **44⅜"**

- Lost **60¾ pounds** of fat in twelve weeks
- Built **5½ pounds** of muscle
- Lost **12⅝"** off waist
- Trimmed **9½"** off thighs

Weeks 3 and 4:

Men: 1,400 calories per day

Women: 1,100 calories per day

Weeks 5 and 6:

Men: 1,300 calories per day

Women: 1,000 calories per day

You'll always have a 300-calorie breakfast, a 300-calorie lunch, and a 300-calorie dinner (women), or a 500-calorie dinner (men). After each two-week period, only your snack calories will change—from 300 to 200 to 100 calories per day (women), or from 400 to 300 to 200 calories per day (men). For each of your five daily meals, you'll have at least three choices.

Everything has been simplified so even the most kitchen-inept man or woman can succeed. Very little cooking is required. All you have to do is read the menus, select your food, and follow directions. It's just that simple!

MENUS FOR WEEKS 1–6

BREAKFAST = 300 CALORIES

Choice of bagel, cereal, or shake.

BAGEL

1 bagel—choice of plain, blueberry, or oat bran—Sara Lee (frozen) (210)

½ ounce light cream cheese (30)

½ cup orange juice, fresh or frozen (55)

Any beverage without calories, caffeine, or sodium, such as decaffeinated coffee or tea

CEREAL

Choice of one: Kellogg's Low-Fat Granola (without raisins), General Mills Honey Nut Clusters, General Mills Basic 4. 1.6 ounces (45 grams) serving equals approximately 170 calories. Weigh the serving on an accurate scale.

½ cup fat-free milk (45)

¾ cup orange juice (82)

Noncaloric beverage

SHAKE (CHOICE OF ONE)

BANANA-ORANGE

1 large banana (8¾" long) (100)

½ cup orange juice (55)

½ cup fat-free milk (45)

2 tablespoons wheat germ (66)

1 teaspoon safflower oil (42)

2 ice cubes (optional)

Place ingredients in blender. Blend until smooth.

CHOCOLATE OR VANILLA

1 packet Carnation Instant Breakfast, or another meal-replacement shake mix, such as Champion Ultramet, Biotest Grow, or EAS Myoplex (you must make appropriate adjustment in serving size), that contains the appropriate calories (110)

1 cup fat-free milk (90)

½ large banana (8¾" long) (50)

1 teaspoon safflower oil (42)

2 ice cubes (optional)

Place ingredients in blender. Blend until smooth.

LUNCH = 300 CALORIES

Choice of sandwich, soup, or chef salad.

SANDWICH

2 slices whole-wheat bread (140)

2 teaspoons Promise Buttery Light Spread (33)

2 ounces white meat (about 8 thin slices from deli)—
chicken or turkey (80)

1 ounce fat-free cheese (1½ slices) (50)

Optional: add 1 teaspoon Dijon mustard to bread (0)

Noncaloric beverage

SOUP

Choice of one: Healthy Choice Hearty Chicken, 15-ounce
can (260), or Campbell's Healthy Request Hearty Vegetable Beef, 16-ounce can (260)

½ slice whole-wheat bread (35)

Noncaloric beverage

CHEF SALAD

2 cups lettuce, chopped (20)

2 ounces white meat—chicken or turkey (80)

2 ounces fat-free cheese (100)

4 slices tomato, chopped (28)

1 tablespoon Italian fat-free dressing (6)

1 slice whole-wheat bread (70)

Noncaloric beverage

MIDAFTERNOON SNACK

Men = 200 calories for weeks 1 and 2; 150 calories for
weeks 3 and 4; 100 calories for weeks 5 and 6.

Women = 150 calories for weeks 1 and 2; 100 calories
for weeks 3 and 4; 50 calories for weeks 5 and 6.

1 large banana (8¾" long) (100)

1 apple (3" diameter) (100)

½ cantaloupe (5" diameter) (94)

5 dried prunes (100)

1 ounce (2 small ½-ounce boxes) raisins (82)

1 cup light, fat-free flavored yogurt (100)

DINNER

Men = 500 calories,

Women = 300 calories

Choice of tuna salad, steak, or frozen microwave meal.

TUNA SALAD DINNER

½ 6-ounce can chunk light tuna in water,
drained (75)

½ cup (4 ounces) whole kernel corn, canned, no salt
added (60)

¼ cup (2 ounces) dark red kidney beans, canned (65)

½ apple, chopped (50)

1 tablespoon Hellmann's Light, Reduced-Calorie
Mayonnaise (50)

1 tablespoon sweet pickle relish (20)

Mix the ingredients in a large bowl.

Noncaloric beverage

Men add:

½ cup sliced white potatoes, canned (45)

2 slices whole-wheat bread (140)

STEAK DINNER

3 ounces lean sirloin, broiled (176)

½ cup sweet peas, canned, no salt added (60)

½ cup sliced beets, canned (35)

½ cup fat-free milk (45)

Noncaloric beverage

Men add:

2 slices whole-wheat bread (140)

1 teaspoon Promise Buttery Light Spread (17)

½ cup fat-free milk (45)

FROZEN MICROWAVE DINNER

Choose one of five recommended meals.

GLAZED CHICKEN, LEAN CUISINE EVERYDAY FAVORITES (230)

⅔ cup fat-free milk (60)

Noncaloric beverage

Men add:

2 slices whole-wheat bread (140)

2 teaspoons Promise Buttery Light Spread (33)

½ cup fat-free milk (45)

VEGETABLE LASAGNA, LEAN CUISINE EVERYDAY FAVORITES (260)

½ cup fat-free milk (45)

Noncaloric beverage

Men add:

2 slices whole-wheat bread (140)

2 teaspoons Promise Buttery Light Spread (33)

½ cup fat-free milk (45)

MACARONI AND CHEESE, WEIGHT WATCHERS (260)

½ cup fat-free milk (45)

Noncaloric beverage

Men add:

2 slices whole-wheat bread (140)

2 teaspoons Promise Buttery Light Spread (33)

½ cup fat-free milk (45)

GRILLED TURKEY BREAST, HEALTHY CHOICE (260)

½ cup skim milk (45)

Noncaloric beverage

Men add:

2 slices whole-wheat bread (140)

2 teaspoons Promise Buttery Light Spread (33)

½ cup fat-free milk (45)

HONEY ROASTED PORK, LEAN CUISINE EVERYDAY FAVORITES (240)

⅔ cup fat-free milk (60)

Noncaloric beverage

Men add:

2 slices whole-wheat bread (140)

2 teaspoons Promise Buttery Light Spread (33)

½ cup fat-free milk (45)

LATE-NIGHT SNACK

Men = 200 calories for weeks 1 and 2; 150 calories for weeks 3 and 4; 100 calories for weeks 5 and 6.

Women = 150 calories for weeks 1 and 2; 100 calories for weeks 3 and 4; 50 calories for weeks 5 and 6.

Choose from afternoon snacks or the following:

½ cup low-fat frozen yogurt (100)

2 cups light microwave popcorn (100)

SHOPPING LIST

The amount of these items you'll shop for will depend on your meal selections. Review your choices and adjust your shopping list accordingly. It might help to photocopy this list each week before doing your shopping.

You should try to have most of the items that follow in your pantry or refrigerator. Having them on hand will reduce your temptation to substitute something that will cause you to break the plan.

STAPLES

Orange juice, fat-free milk, whole-wheat bread (make sure first ingredient is 100 percent whole wheat), Promise Buttery Light Spread, Italian fat-free dressing, Dijon mustard, safflower oil, noncaloric beverages (decaffeinated coffee and tea, diet soft drinks, water).

GRAINS

Bagels—choice of plain, blueberry, or oat bran— Sara Lee (frozen), cereals—choice of Kellogg's Low-Fat Granola (without raisins), General Mills Honey Nut Clusters, General Mills Basic 4, wheat germ, popcorn (microwave light).

FRUITS

Bananas, large (8¾" long), apples (3" diameter), cantaloupes (5" diameter), dried prunes, raisins.

VEGETABLES

Lettuce, tomatoes, whole kernel corn (canned, no salt added), sweet peas (canned, no salt added), sliced white potatoes (canned), sliced beets (canned), dark red kidney beans (canned).

DAIRY

Yogurt (light fat-free), cream cheese (light), cheese (fat-free), low-fat frozen yogurt, Carnation Instant Breakfast packets (or something similar).

MEAT, POULTRY, FISH, AND ENTRÉES

Chicken (thin sliced), turkey (thin sliced), tuna (canned in water), sirloin steak (lean).

CANNED SOUP

Campbell's Healthy Request Hearty Vegetable Beef, Healthy Choice Hearty Chicken.

FROZEN MICROWAVE DINNERS OR ENTRÉES

Lean Cuisine Everyday Favorites: Glazed Chicken, Vegetable Lasagna, Honey Roasted Pork; Weight Watchers Macaroni and Cheese; Healthy Choice Grilled Turkey Breast. (*Note:* Frozen food products, especially microwave dinners, are sometimes changed or discontinued. If a menu item is not available in your area, substitute a similar product.)

WHAT'S NEXT

The success of the Body-Leanness Plan is based on a dynamic formula:

• An intense *strength-training routine* that involves moving smoothly against the resistance supplied by a Bowflex machine.

• A simple *eating plan* that emphasizes basic foods and gradually reduces calories.

• A synergizing *superhydration schedule* that accelerates building muscle and losing fat.

This dynamic formula is important throughout the other chapters in Part IV. It remains important, with some modifications, through chapters 27 and 28, which are concerned with maintenance and follow-up. Also, you'll want to investigate chapter 29, since many of the answers to the frequently asked questions will help you combat potential problems.

21
THE HARD-BODY CHALLENGE:

A SIX-WEEK, GET-RIPPED COURSE
FOR ATHLETES

I HAD A TOUGH TIME BELIEVING WHAT I was seeing. I was at Sea World's Bayside Stadium in Orlando in May of 2001, watching the water-ski team perform. Peter Fleck, a champion skier and corporate show director of World Entertainment, had invited me to be his guest.

Granted, the performances were outstanding and the skills—from barefooting to jumping to adagio—were awesome. What I had a difficult time accepting was how *soft* some of the guys looked.

Don't get me wrong. They were in above-average shape compared to the normal population. What they lacked, however, was that *ripped, tight, muscular appearance* that some highly conditioned athletes attain prior to competition.

Why was having that ripped, muscular look so important in my mind? Because leaner bodies perform more efficiently, are more resistant to injury, and *look better*.

Looking better seemed especially important because at the end of each Sea World show, the water-skiers assemble at center stage on the lakefront to sign autographs and be photographed with the spectators. There are few things more impressionable, for both youngsters and adults, than to be up close and photographed with well-built athletes in swim-suits.

"What kind of training program are these guys on?" I asked Fleck as we were walking to the parking lot. "I didn't see a really defined man in the group. Don't these guys realize how much better they'd look and perform with less fat and leaner, harder bodies?"

"They're still suffering from the winter bloat," he replied. "You know how difficult it is to stay in shape with all the socializing during the holidays."

I knew what Fleck was talking about. Approximately 70 percent of the adult population in the United States gains from 3 to 5 pounds of body fat each year from Thanksgiving through the Super Bowl. I just wasn't aware that these statistics also applied to professional water-skiers at Sea World. Plus, the holiday season had been over for almost four months!

Peter and I both agreed that something needed to be done to motivate the Sea World guys into action. Because of my continuing interest in research on fat loss, I told him that if he could arrange a meeting, I'd be happy to develop and implement a program specifically for their water-skiers.

BOWFLEX CALLING

Later that afternoon, I received a phone call from Randy Potter, chief operating officer of the parent company of Bowflex. He mentioned that he wanted me to do some field-testing on a new Bowflex machine called the Ultimate. In fact, he had two of them packaged and ready to ship to me the next day. "Do you," he wanted to know, "have any overfat people in the Orlando area who I could supervise through a six-week eating and exercising program?"

"Funny you should ask," I replied. When Potter heard the idea, he was fully supportive. He could already see the benefits of muscular water-skiers training on Bowflex. Furthermore, Potter noted that Bowflex was testing a new line of engineered food products for use in weight loss in 2002. He said he would also supply nutritious shake packets and energy bars for the athletes.

The next day I called Fleck and we came up with a solid plan. I would organize the eating and exercising routine, and he would get approval from Sea World to house the Bowflex Ultimate machine in Bayside Stadium. Then, he would call a meeting for all interested water-skiers where we would introduce the pro-

gram, explain what was involved, and issue what I called the Hard-Body Challenge.

The objective of the Hard-Body Challenge was to get the guys dissatisfied with their soft bodies and motivated to take action. My job was to establish a fat-loss goal for each participant and, most important, to help them reach their goals in six weeks or less.

Five members of the men's water-ski team at Sea World accepted the challenge. I met with them two days later to take each participant's body weight, skin fold/body-fat percentage, circumference measurements, and full-body photographs in a bathing suit. I also went over what was expected of each participant.

THREE COMPONENTS FOR SUCCESS

Success of the program was based primarily on my three-part formula: reduced-calorie eating, strength training, and superhydration.

The course started on July 15, 2001, and finished on August 26, 2001. Each man, I'm pleased to report, reached his goal. Tom Wykle did the best by dropping 35 pounds of fat and $5\frac{3}{8}$ inches off his waist. The least amount lost was $15\frac{1}{2}$ pounds by

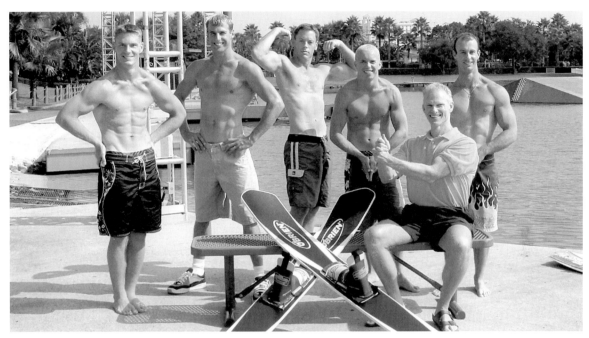

The Hard-Body Team from Sea World in Orlando lost 120 pounds of fat in only six weeks. From left to right: Tom Wykle, Gary Smith, Dan Justman, Sharky Anderson, Ellington Darden (seated), and Darin Truttmann.

THE MUCH-ADMIRED 32-INCH WAIST

Twenty years ago, a 32-inch waist was what every man trying to get in shape wanted. It was a much-admired trademark of vim, vigor, and virility. Today, a fitness-minded man still wants a 32-inch waist, but he also strives for a six-pack abdominal formation etched upon the front of his midsection. For the abdominal muscles to show clearly through the skin, a man must have a very low percentage of body fat.

Since there is much emphasis on the waistline in our culture, I often take circumference measurements of the midsection at three levels: 2 inches above the navel, at the navel, and 2 inches below the navel. I've found that

some men tend to lose fat first from the navel area. Others lose it above the navel, then the navel, and finally from below the navel. A few start from below and work upward. These three slightly different measurements provide insight into the fat-ordering process.

Interestingly, the water-skiers dropped the most from the navel area: 4 inches. They went from an average of 34.675 inches *before*, to 30.675 inches *after*. At the end of the study, each of the water-skiers had not a 32-inch waist but a 31-inch waist, as well as a muscular six-pack.

Congratulations, guys, on a job well done.

Darin Truttmann, who was also the most muscular of the men at the start. Darin accomplished his goal in only three weeks.

AVERAGE WEIGHT AND FAT LOST

Men (N = 5)	Before	After	Difference
Body weight (lbs.)	188.0	167.0	21.0
Percent body fat	17.1	5.3	11.8
Pounds of fat	32.2	8.8	23.4

Note: The men had an average age of 27.8 years and an average height of 71.2 inches.

AVERAGE INCHES LOST

Circumference Site	Men (N = 5)
2 inches above navel	3.6
Navel	4.0
2 inches below navel	3.2
Hips	3.1
Right thigh	2.0
Left thigh	2.0
Total inches lost	17.9

THE HARD-BODY CHALLENGE

Let's face it, many athletes and fitness-minded men and women may gain some excess fat at times. We all tend to relax occasionally during the year and get a little soft. If that's the case with you, then the Hard-Body Challenge will do the job. The Hard-Body Challenge is different from the Body-Leanness Plan because it is geared for athletes who are already in above-average shape. Consequently, the recommended calories per day are significantly higher, and they do not decrease.

If you are already a well-conditioned individual but have added a few pounds, now is the time to learn more about the components of the Hard-Body Challenge and then make a commitment to it.

REDUCED-CALORIE EATING

The cornerstone of any successful fat-loss program must involve eating fewer calories. It's a scientific fact that in losing fat, *calories do count.*

Surveys reveal that young men in the United States eat from 3,000 to 4,000 calories per day. During the holiday season, and other times of the year, many regularly exceed that amount. The Sea World skiers were all regularly eating too many calories on most days.

An eating plan of slightly below 2,000 calories a day for active young men seemed to be a level that

TOM WYKLE'S RESULTS

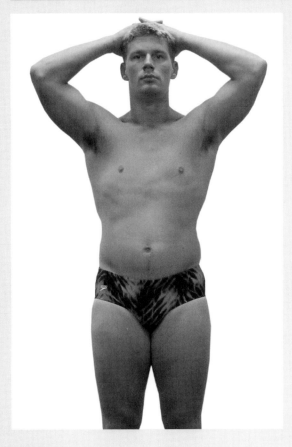 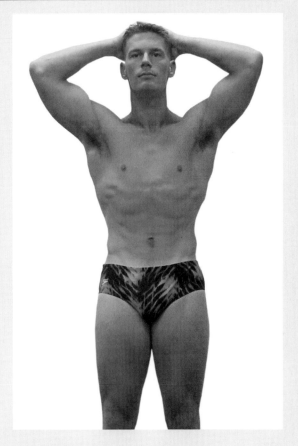

AGE: **28**
HEIGHT: **6'1"**
BEFORE WEIGHT: **223¾ POUNDS**
BEFORE WAIST SIZE: **37¼"**

- Lost **35½ pounds** of fat in six weeks
- Built **3¾ pounds** of muscle
- Trimmed **5½"** off waist

was just right for efficient fat loss. Thus, each water-skier's calories were reduced from 3,000 or more per day to 1,900. (*Note:* active women applying the program should lower their calories to 1,500 per day. See the Hard-Body Menus on the following page for specific details.)

Besides eating fewer calories, *smaller meals* can help cut the fat. The idea is to plan six small meals a day, never going longer than three hours between meals. This helps you feel more satiated and less hungry throughout your waking hours.

Please examine the menus that follow. Calories for each food are listed in parentheses. The midmorning, midafternoon, and evening snacks are comprised of Champion Nutrition supplements: Ultramet, a high-protein shake mix, and SnacBar, a high-protein energy bar. (*Note:* If Champion products are not available in your nutrition store, you may substitute other shake mixes and energy bars with similar calorie counts.) The other meals are made from foods available in any local supermarket.

HARD-BODY MENUS

Men: 1,900 calories per day

Women: 1,500 calories per day

From the menus below, women should subtract the following: 1 medium-size fruit (80) from Midmorning Snack, 1 Champion SnacBar (180) from Midafternoon Snack, 1 slice whole-grain bread (70) from Dinner, and 1 medium-size fruit (80) from Evening Snack.

BREAKFAST = 400 CALORIES

1 bagel, Lender's New York Style, frozen, toasted (250)

1 slice processed Swiss cheese (70)

¾ cup orange juice (83)

Noncaloric beverage

MIDMORNING SNACK = 220 CALORIES

½ Champion Ultramet packet mixed with 7 ounces cold water (140)

1 medium-sized fruit (apple, orange, banana, or 1 ounce raisins) (80)

LUNCH = 400 CALORIES

SANDWICH

2 slices whole-grain bread (140)

1 tablespoon light mayonnaise (50)

3 ounces white meat chicken or turkey (120)

1 tablespoon sweet pickle relish (20)

2 tomato slices (14)

Noncaloric beverage

MIDAFTERNOON SNACK = 260 CALORIES

1 Champion SnacBar (180)

1 medium-sized fruit (apple, orange, banana, or 1 ounce raisins) (80)

DINNER = 400 CALORIES

Choice of tuna salad or one of three frozen microwave meals.

SHARKY ANDERSON'S RESULTS

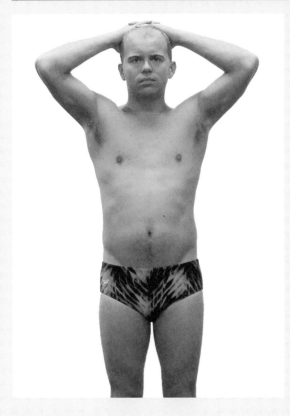
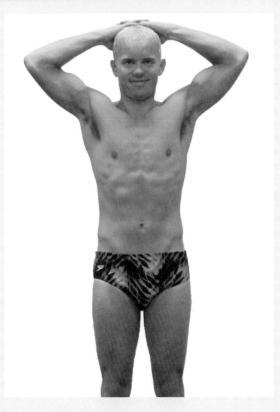

AGE: **24**

HEIGHT: **5'9"**

BEFORE WEIGHT: **161 POUNDS**

BEFORE WAIST SIZE: **34½"**

- Lost **21 pounds** of fat in six weeks
- Built **2½ pounds** of muscle
- Trimmed **4¾"** off waist

TUNA SALAD DINNER

½ 6-ounce can chunk light tuna in water, drained (75)

½ cup (4 ounces) whole kernel corn, canned, no salt added (60)

¼ cup (2 ounces) dark red kidney beans, canned (65)

1 tablespoon sweet pickle relish (20)

1 tablespoon light mayonnaise (50)

2 slices whole-grain bread (140)

Mix the ingredients in a large bowl.

Noncaloric beverage

FROZEN MICROWAVE DINNERS

Choose one of three recommended meals.

BLACKENED CHICKEN, HEALTHY CHOICE (320)

1 slice whole-grain bread (70)

Noncaloric beverage

GLAZED TURKEY TENDERLOINS, LEAN CUISINE CAFÉ
CLASSICS (260)

2 slices whole-grain bread (140)

Noncaloric beverage

LASAGNA WITH MEAT SAUCE, MICHELINA'S AUTHENTICO
(290)

1½ slices whole-grain bread (105)

Noncaloric beverage

EVENING SNACK = 220 CALORIES

½ Champion Ultramet packet mixed with 7 ounces of cold
water (140)

1 medium-size fruit (apple, orange, banana, or 1 ounce
raisins) (80)

Notes: Noncaloric beverages are any type of water,
soft drink, tea, or coffee with zero calories and no caffeine. Whole-grain bread—try to select a bread that
lists as the first ingredient whole, sprouted, or cracked
grain. Other frozen microwave meals may be substituted for those listed. Select one that has from 250 to
320 calories and no more than 5 to 7 grams of fat.

STRENGTH TRAINING

Reduced-calorie eating alone does produce weight
loss. But in almost all cases, some of that weight
loss comes from the muscles. Losing weight from
your muscles is a critical concern. It makes you
weaker and causes your performance to suffer. This
cannot occur for long-term success, and it's certainly
not recommended for athletes who practice and perform multiple times each week. The ideal condition
is to lose weight *only* from your fat stores.

For this to occur, you have to strengthen your muscles at the same time that you reduce your calories.
Strength training prevents the loss of fluids from
your muscles. In fact, strength training can actually
build from ½ to 1 pound of muscle per week. For this
to happen, however, the exercise must be done intensely and progressively.

In the routines that follow, the same ones I recommended for the Sea World water-skiers, do one set of
between 8 and 12 repetitions on each exercise. When
you can perform 12 or more repetitions of an exercise, make a written note on your workout card found
on page 285. Then, on the following workout, increase
the resistance by 10 pounds. On a Bowflex machine,
that means adding a 5-pound Power Rod to each side.

Such an increase will usually reduce your repetitions to 8 or 9. It's now your goal to add a repetition each workout until 12 or more are accomplished, and the progression is continued again and again.

Training on three nonconsecutive days per week provides your body with the needed consistency and ample recovery time. Monday-Wednesday-Friday schedules are usually preferred, as was the case with the Sea World athletes.

HARD-BODY
STRENGTH-TRAINING ROUTINES

WEEKS 1 AND 2

1. Leg Curl

2. Leg Extension

3. Bench Press

4. Standing Biceps Curl

5. Lying Shoulder Pullover

6. Triceps Pushdown

7. Seated Abdominal Crunch

WEEKS 3 AND 4

1. Leg Curl

2. Leg Extension

3. Chest Fly*

4. Bench Press

5. Biceps Curl

6. Reverse Grip Pulldown*

7. Triceps Pushdown

8. Seated Abdominal Crunch

* New exercise

During Weeks 3 and 4, eliminate the Lying Shoulder Pullover and add the Chest Fly and the Reverse Grip Pulldown. Your total exercises per workout are now eight.

WEEKS 5 AND 6

1. Leg Curl

2. Leg Extension

3. Leg Press*

4. Chest Fly

5. Biceps Curl

6. Reverse Grip Pulldown

7. Triceps Pushdown

8. Reverse Curl*

9. Seated Abdominal Crunch

*New exercise

DAN JUSTMAN'S RESULTS

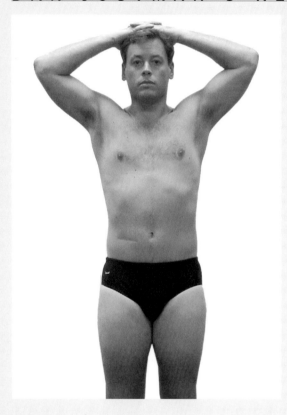 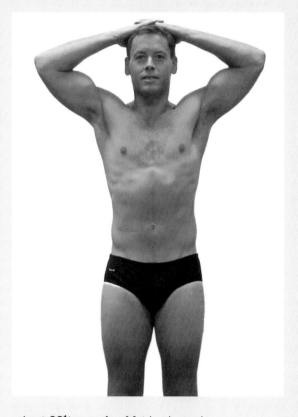

AGE: **29**

HEIGHT: **6'2"**

BEFORE WEIGHT: **202½ POUNDS**

BEFORE WAIST SIZE: **35"**

- Lost **28½ pounds** of fat in six weeks
- Built **5 pounds** of muscle
- Trimmed **4⅛"** off waist

The routine for Weeks 5 and 6 removes the Bench Press and adds the Leg Press and Reverse Curl. There are now nine exercises to do three times per week.

SUPERHYDRATION

The superhydration schedule is exactly the same as the one outlined on page 177. Review the guidelines and follow them precisely.

MAINTENANCE GUIDELINES

How do you know if you've lost all of your excess fat? One way is to recall what it felt like to be in the best shape of your life. Perhaps, for example, it was when you were in high school. Remember what you weighed then, as well as your waist size. Attaining those numbers may be an indication that your excess fat has been removed.

Since I was working with athletes in this particular study, the goal for each water-skier was to lower his body fat from an average of 17 percent to 6 percent. From my experience, 6 percent is a healthy level to attain. Unless you are planning to compete in a body-building contest, there is no advantage to going below this level. Four of the five water-skiers successfully reached 6 percent or lower, and the other finished in the 8-percent range.

Once you are satisfied with your level of body fat, the objective changes from weight *loss* to weight *maintenance*. Successful maintenance requires a continuation of the practices initiated over the previous six weeks, with some minor adjustments. More about maintenance is covered in chapter 28.

GET SERIOUS!

Dan Justman, who lost nearly 29 pounds of fat and 4 inches off his waist, said it best: "Before the program, I was sort of walking around in an eating and exercising limbo. The Hard-Body Challenge opened my eyes—and made me finally get serious."

You, too, need to *open your eyes—and finally get serious*. Accept the Hard-Body Challenge now.

With disciplined application of the Hard-Body guidelines, you'll be leaner, stronger, and more muscular *in six weeks or less!*

22
HIPS & THIGHS—
TACKLING THE TOUGH SPOTS:

A SIX-WEEK LOWER-BODY COURSE FOR WOMEN

FOR MANY WOMEN, THE BATTLE of the bulge starts and ends with the hips and thighs. "If only my hips matched the rest of me," one woman remarked to me several years ago. "If I could just tighten my thunder thighs," another woman sighed. Both of these women joined one of my six-week courses in Dallas and surprised themselves by achieving great results on traditional tough spots.

Yes, hips and thighs—from many a woman's point of view—are areas of major concern. These fat-laden body parts often withstand many novel exercises and dozens of exotic diets with no noticeable change in their appearance. If you've always had a problem with your hips and thighs, or perhaps only recently noticed laxity and flabbiness in these body parts, then this six-week course will help solve your problem. First, let's discuss why women store fat around their hips and thighs.

THE HIPS AND THIGHS: FAVORITES FOR FAT STORAGE

Why do women have more fat than men and, in particular, thicker layers around their hips and thighs? The simple answer is female hormones, but a more complete answer comes from an understanding of puberty, menstruation, and pregnancy.

Puberty. There is minimum difference of body-fat levels between the sexes in childhood. At puberty, however, girls begin depositing fat and boys start putting on muscle. A young girl, in fact, must have approximately 15 to 20 percent of her weight as fat before she can start to menstruate.

Menstruation. Both sexes produce hormones that make them male or female. For women, the two primary hormones are estrogen and progesterone. Both can contribute to fatness.

The interacting rise and fall of estrogen and progesterone regulates a woman's menstrual cycle. The same estrogen that is involved in your menstrual cycle also causes you to deposit fat in your breasts, hips, buttocks, and thighs. It does this by chemically stimulating cells in those areas to store fat.

Progesterone jumps in by affecting your appetite and mood. It makes you hungrier during the second half of your menstrual cycle and is also responsible for the ravenous appetite that many women have during pregnancy. Progesterone can also make you feel sluggish, sleepy, and less inclined to exercise.

Pregnancy. Research shows that the average weight gain from the beginning of the first trimester until the end of pregnancy is 27.5 pounds, of which about 20 percent is fat. Progesterone levels stay high from the beginning of pregnancy to the end. But progesterone is not the real culprit when it comes to weight gain during pregnancy. That distinction belongs to the fat cells.

Fat cells can multiply during periods of rapid weight gain, such as infancy and puberty. But with pregnancy, women often add fat cells in a way that men never have to endure. Further pregnancies tend to complicate the situation, since once a fat cell has been formed it stays forever, always demanding to be filled. This is the primary reason most of the fat gained during pregnancy tends to hang on so tenaciously, long after the baby is born.

Wide hips also help women during pregnancy. Women with a natural tendency to deposit fat over their upper thighs have an easier time giving birth than women with thin hips.

THERE'S HOPE: YOU'RE NOT FATED TO BE FAT!

Extra fat around the hips and thighs of most women is a biological fact of life and one that was programmed into the species long ago by nature. Maybe you are a woman who has inherited a larger-than-average number of fat cells around your hips and thighs. Regardless of the number, fat cells can shrink. You can still lose pounds and inches from your lower body.

Depending on your genetics, however, you may have a harder time getting lean than other women. If that's the case, you'll deal with the fact best by facing it head-on and realizing that you'll require extra time and effort to overcome it. If you want great hips and thighs badly enough, no roadblocks will stop you. You're not fated to be fat—absolutely not!

Before moving into the actual program, there's another concept that needs to be addressed: *cellulite.*

THE REAL FACTS ABOUT CELLULITE

Here are the facts: Cellulite is subcutaneous adipose tissue just like any common body fat. Since most women have thick layers of fat directly under the skin on their upper thighs and buttocks, it appears there first. The rippled effect is caused by the fibers of connective tissue in the area, which lose their elasticity with age. The overlying skin attached to these fibers then contracts. If the size of the encased fat does not

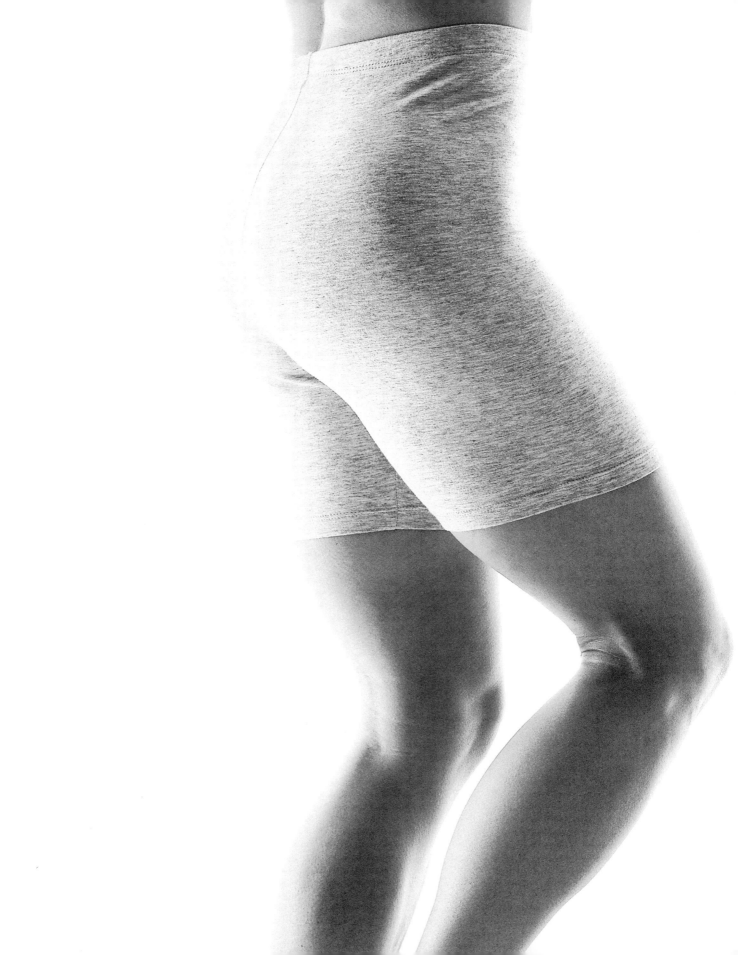

shrink proportionately, a dimpling occurs on the surface of the skin.

Unfortunately, there are no quick-and-easy solutions to removing dimpled fatty deposits on the hips and thighs. *All fat, regardless of the location and the thickness, is difficult to remove.* Fat cannot be massaged, perspired, relaxed, soaked, flushed, compressed, or dissolved out of the body.

As I noted in chapter 13, to get rid of fat from your body, heat energy has to be transferred gradually through your skin, lungs, and urine into the environment. There are no other ways—PERIOD.

The most complete treatment for dimpled fatty deposits, cellulite, flab, or anything else fat is what I've been discussing throughout this book:

• You must reduce the size of the subcutaneous fat cells.

• You must increase the size and strength of the underlying muscles, especially those of the hips and thighs.

This six-week course does both.

THE LOWER-BODY PROGRAM

The lower-body program consists of an eating plan, superhydration, and a Bowflex strength-training routine. The eating plan is exactly the same as the diet in chapter 20. The superhydration schedule for this chapter is identical to the one in chapter 19. The Bowflex workouts are specifically designed for tackling the trouble spots: the hips and thighs.

Let's examine the major points of the program.

LOWER-BODY EATING PLAN

Please turn back to chapter 20, page 187, to review the details of the eating plan. During the six-week program, you always have a 300-calorie breakfast, lunch, and dinner. That will not change. What will change are your snack calories. Your snack calories will decrease with each two-week segment: from 300 to 200 to 100 calories. Your total calories per day will be:

1,200 calories for Weeks 1 and 2

1,100 calories for Weeks 3 and 4

1,000 calories for Weeks 5 and 6

SUPERHYDRATION

Superhydration is an important aspect of reducing the fatty deposits from your hips and thighs. I recommend that you follow the schedule on page 177.

Notice that the water drinking is progressive. You begin by sipping four 32-ounce containers of ice-cold water a day. During week 6 you'll be up to six-and-a-half bottles a day. That seems like a lot of water—and it is. But don't worry. Thousands of women have superhydrated in the same way. It won't take you long to realize the advantages of keeping your system well hydrated.

STRENGTH TRAINING FOR THE HIPS AND THIGHS

There is no exercise, or group of exercises, that effectively reduces fat from only your hips and thighs. The next chapter explains why spot reduction of fat is impossible, but while spot reduction is not possible, spot production of muscle is not only possible, but recommended.

Remember, the solution to eliminating cellulite has two parts. First, you must shrink your body's fat cells, most of which will probably come from your lower body. Shrinking these fat cells eases the stress on the connective tissue. Second, you must increase the size and strength of the large muscles that compose the hips and thighs. Thicker muscle, unlike fat, is rigid, and rigidity smoothes the overlying fat, connective tissue, and skin.

The idea is to lose fat and build muscle *simultaneously* in your hips and thighs. Accomplishing this goal will help considerably with the problem.

Next, most women will benefit from counterbalancing their hips and thighs by strength-training certain body parts. Counterbalancing in the design world is achieved by taking attention away from a focal point and moving the emphasis in another direction. You probably remember the fashion trend of the 1980s that featured broad shoulders by placing padding in women's dresses, jackets, and even T-shirts. Well, you can do something similar by strength-training your shoulder muscles. Broader shoulders counterbalance your hips and thighs.

Lastly, shapely calves—just like broad shoulders—can divert attention away from dominant hips and thighs. So at least one exercise in your routine should involve your calves.

Here are the Bowflex routines that I recommend for the six-week course. I add two exercises after each two-week segment. Do one set of 8 to 12 repetitions on all exercises, except for the Wall Squat, which is a new movement that I'll describe for Weeks 3 and 4. Practice the routine three times per week on alternating days. The proper form for each of the exercises is covered in chapters 6–8. Refer to those chapters if you have difficulty performing any of the exercises.

Note: Perform the bracketed exercises with minimal rest in between.

JANE KNUTH'S RESULTS

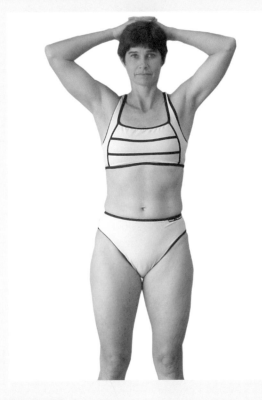 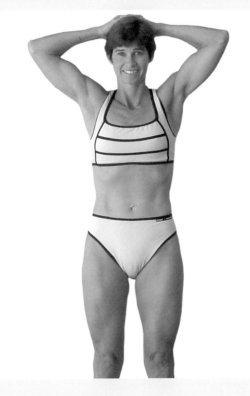

AGE: **40**

HEIGHT: **5'9"**

BEFORE WEIGHT: **150½ POUNDS**

BEFORE WAIST SIZE: **29¼"**

- Lost **19¼ pounds** of fat in six weeks
- Built **3 pounds** of muscle
- Trimmed **2⅞"** off waist
- Eliminated **3¼"** off hips
- Dropped **4¼"** off thighs

WEEKS 1 AND 2: HIP AND THIGH ROUTINE

1. Leg Curl

2. Leg Extension

3. Seated Calf Raise

4. Standing Lateral Raise

5. Seated Shoulder Press

6. Seated Abdominal Crunch

7. Leg Press

WEEKS 3 AND 4: HIP AND THIGH ROUTINE

1. Leg Curl

2. Leg Extension

3. Wall Squat with Static Hold*

4. Seated Calf Raise

5. Standing Lateral Raise

6. Seated Shoulder Press

7. Reverse Grip Pulldown*

8. Seated Abdominal Crunch

9. Leg Press

*New exercise

During weeks 3 and 4, your routine includes two new exercises—the Reverse Grip Pulldown and the Wall Squat with Static Hold, which is performed immediately after the Leg Extension and does not require a Bowflex machine. It's a freehand exercise that involves only a smooth wall. Here's how to do it.

Wall Squat with Static Hold: Stand erect and lean back against a smooth, sturdy wall. Position your heels shoulder width apart and approximately 12 inches away from the base of the wall. Place your hands on top of your head and slide your back down the wall until the tops of your thighs are parallel to the floor. Now is when the exercise begins. Hold this 90-degree, bent-kneed position statically (with almost no movement) for at least 30 seconds, until you finally have to slide down and sit on the floor. Stabilize yourself on the floor and carefully stand up.

That's it. Just one static-hold repetition for 30 seconds. But wait—that's just the first session. Each subsequent workout, you must add 5 seconds to your hold time. By the end of the course, your static-hold time will be 90 seconds, or very near it.

You're going to like this simple little exercise; well, maybe not the way it burns your thighs while you're doing it, but the thigh-firming results you'll achieve from it.

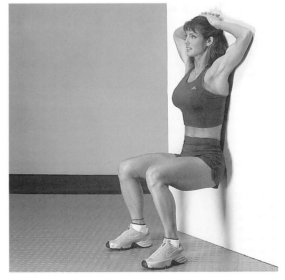

Wall Squat with Static Hold: Breathe frequently as you hold this position for 30 seconds or more.

KARI FLECK'S RESULTS

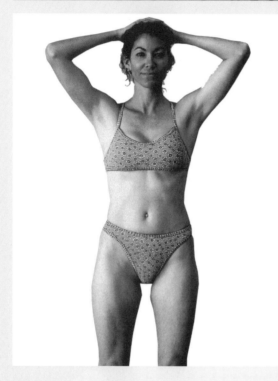 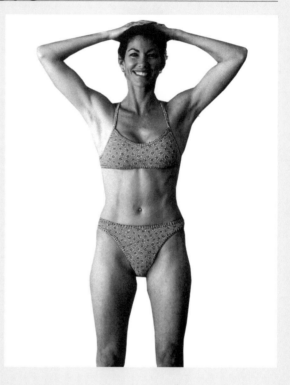

AGE: **34**

HEIGHT: **5'8"**

BEFORE WEIGHT: **122½ POUNDS**

BEFORE WAIST SIZE: **27⅛"**

- Lost **9 pounds** of fat in six weeks
- Built **1 pound** of muscle
- Trimmed **1¼"** off waist
- Dropped **1⅝"** off thighs

WEEKS 5 AND 6: HIP AND THIGH ROUTINE

1. Leg Curl

2. Leg Extension

3. Wall Squat with Static Hold

4. Seated Calf Raise

5. Standing Lateral Raise

6. Seated Shoulder Press

7. Reverse Grip Pulldown

8. Seated Abdominal Crunch

9. Leg Press

10. Seated Leg Curl*

11. Wide Wall Squat with Static Hold*

*New exercise

Remember the pre-exhaustion technique from chapter 10? That's where one exercise fatigues some of the same muscles that you're using in a second and even third exercise. Performing two or three exercises, back to back, with no more than 5 seconds between movements, allows you to make a greater inroad into your existing strength level.

To get the full effect from the routine of weeks 5 and 6, it's best to involve pre-exhaustion and move quickly between exercises 1, 2, and 3—and exercises 9, 10, and 11. It can be a little hectic between these exercises, and having assistance to adjust the Power Rods will help.

Two new exercises are added during this segment. I rarely advocate doing two sets of the same exercise during the same workout, but both of the new exercises are similar to exercises you're already performing. The Seated Leg Curl contributes a different feel, because of the hip-flexion involvement, to your hamstrings. The Wide Wall Squat with Static Hold is similar to the previously described Wall Squat.

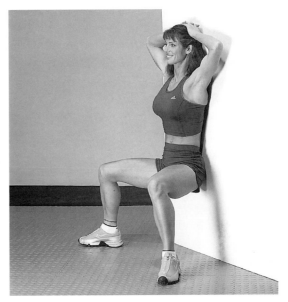

Wide Wall Squat with Static Hold: Position your heels approximately 30 inches apart and make sure that the tops of your thighs remain parallel to the floor.

Wide Wall Squat with Static Hold: Get into the same position as before with one modification: Place each foot 8 to 10 inches wider so that there are approximately 30 inches between your heels. A wide-squat position involves more of the inner-thigh, adductor muscle group than a narrow-squat stance. Slide down the wall, make sure the tops of your thighs are parallel to the floor, and hold statically for 30 seconds. Add 5 seconds or more holding time to each of your next five sessions, and try to progress up to 60 seconds. Once again, you're going to really feel this movement.

Stay focused, push down with your heels, relax your face, and breathe repeatedly. You can do it!

TACKLING THOSE TOUGH SPOTS

This program provides you with the strength and stamina that you need to tackle those tough spots: your hips and thighs. The eating plan, superhydration, and the specific Bowflex routines zero in on the major requirements for losing fat and building muscle. Of course, you also want to include as many of the other factors mentioned in earlier chapters as you possibly can for better and faster results.

Finally, don't be afraid of building excessively large muscles in your lower body. It's not likely to happen—unless you have rare inherited characteristics. Such a woman would have to have unusually short tendons and long muscle bellies. (Most muscles have a teardrop shape; the large middle is called the belly. Thus, a long-bellied muscle would look more like a football than a teardrop.) This combination is rare even among men. Only one person in a million inherits these traits.

In spite of these seldom-seen genetic traits, many women still worry about overdeveloping their lower-body muscles—primarily the gluteals, quadriceps, hamstrings, and gastrocnemius and soleus. Larger muscles, in fact, are the very thing needed for better legs.

LARGER MUSCLES: AN ASSET

Some of the best legs I've ever seen belonged to Brenda Harris, a mechanical engineer who worked at the Nautilus headquarters in Dallas from 1987 to 1990. Even though Harris had been involved in various forms of exercise for many years, her fear was that strength training would make her legs overly large. After lengthy discussions, she finally agreed to go through one of my six-week programs.

Over the next month and a half, Harris added 5.13 pounds of muscle to her 5 foot 6 inch, 120-pound body. In the process she reduced her body fat to 14.6 percent—and her great legs became *even better*.

If you ever do develop a muscle that is too large, all you have to do is stop exercising it. Within a week, the muscle begins to atrophy, or lose size from disuse.

So you really do want larger muscles. Larger muscles are your ticket to drop pounds and firm flab. They are the key—not only to tackling your trouble spots but to reversing the muscle loss process.

With the Bowflex strength-training routines, you can help create the hips and thighs that you've always wanted—with less fat and more muscle.

The power is yours *still!*

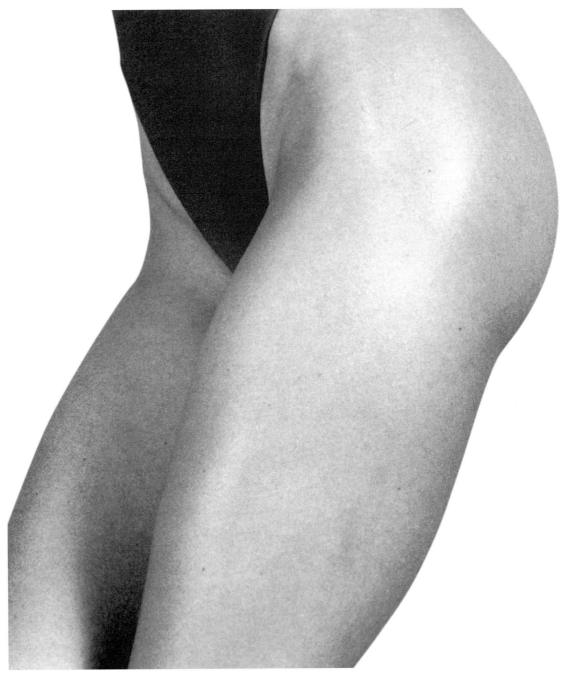

After adding more than 5 pounds of muscle to her body, Brenda Harris's hips and thighs could be classified as awesome.

23

ABDOMINAL FOCUS:

A SIX-WEEK COURSE
FOR A FLATTER STOMACH

THIS COURSE WAS DESIGNED FOR MY friend Peter Fleck, the corporate show director at World Entertainment and the leader of the Orlando Sea World water-ski team. When I met him in the spring of 2001, I thought he would be an excellent candidate for the Hard-Body Challenge. Prior business endeavors, however, made it impossible for him to join. As the study progressed and the guys' strength and muscularity started showing, I could tell Fleck wished he had been one of the participants.

After the completion of the study, Fleck, who was now more motivated than ever to get in tip-top shape, kept touching base with me—hoping we could organize another group of overfat subjects to train on Bowflex. Different commitments always prevented us from following through. His enthusiasm, however, did not wane, and neither did his waistline.

pect he expected that I would jump up halfway through the evening and, just like Mickey Rooney in those old Andy Hardy movies, announce, "Hey gang, I've got a great idea. After the holidays, let's organize a new fat-loss project!"

Actually, I had a nice time meeting his friends, who had many other interests besides losing weight. But, yes, early in 2002, I did organize a small group, which included Fleck, to go through a six-week course that centered around removing fat from the midsection.

Peter was the leader of the pack. He reduced his body fat from 17.4 to 5.9 percent by losing 24 pounds of fat and 4¼ inches off his waist. At the end of the program, he had some of the most defined abdominal muscles that I've ever seen on an athlete. See for yourself on page 227.

PARTY TIME

Skip forward four months; it's the Christmas season and I've been invited to a party where I will see Peter and his wife, Kari. I'm unaware that he has invited a select group of his middle-aged, fat friends. And he had already told them what I do in hopes of making weight loss a discussion topic. Knowing Fleck, I sus-

BEING REALISTIC

If you've got a problem with excessive belly fat, then this program is for you. If you simply want a flatter stomach, then this program is for you. If you want rippling abdominal muscles that resemble Peter Fleck's—and you have genetics similar to his—then this program is also for you.

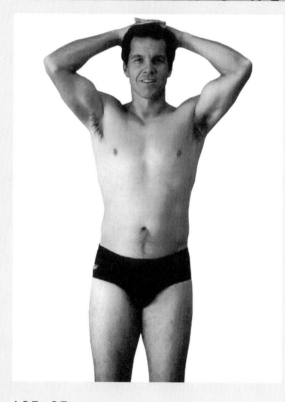 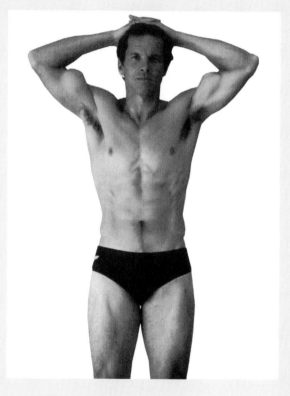

AGE: **37**

HEIGHT: **6'1"**

BEFORE WEIGHT: **197 POUNDS**

BEFORE WAIST SIZE: **34⅞"**

- Lost **24 pounds** of fat in six weeks
- Built **2 pounds** of muscle
- Trimmed **4¼"** off waist
- Dropped **4⅞"** off thighs

Fleck has dark hair, dark eyes, and height, which give him an advantage in achieving extreme leanness. Without the correct genes, you may never have rippling abdominals, but you can certainly improve the muscularity of your midsection, as long as you're realistic.

THE TRUTH
ABOUT SPOT REDUCTION

Spot reduction is the idea that by exercising a specific body part, such as the abdominals, you can burn off the fat surrounding those muscles. This belief is the reason high-repetition sit-ups, leg raises, and twisting movements have been practiced for years as a way to remove fat from the waist. Such beliefs and practices, however, are not based on science.

The fat that is stored around your waist exists in a form called lipids. To be used as energy, the lipids must first be converted to fatty acids. This is a very complex chemical procedure that occurs after the lipids travel through the bloodstream to the liver. After being converted to fatty acids, they are then transported to the working muscles as fuel. Spot reduction would make sense if the fat cells selected to be converted into fuel were from the areas where you have the thickest layers of fat, but this does not happen. There are no direct pathways from the fat cells to the muscle cells.

When fat is used for energy, it comes through the liver from fat cells located all over the body. Which cells your body uses first is genetically programmed. Generally, it occurs in reverse order from where you most recently stored fat; that is, the last places you stored fat are the first from which you lose it.

Consequently, spot reduction of fat is physiologically impossible. Those people recommending or performing specific spot-reducing exercises are misinformed. Interestingly, even if spot reduction of body fat were possible, abdominal exercises do not burn very many calories. For example, an average man who performs 60 seconds of abdominal crunches or sit-ups burns only 7.5 calories. At the rate of 7.5 calories per minute, it would take 7 hours and 47 minutes of continuous repetitions (at 10 per minute that's 4,660 repetitions) to get rid of 3,500 calories, or 1 pound of fat. That is not exactly what I'd call efficiency in action!

But while spot reduction is not possible, spot gains of strength in certain body parts is. Isolating and strengthening the muscles in your midsection can automatically decrease your waistline, even if no attention is given to reducing your calories. That's one advantage of spot-specific Bowflex exercises.

WHAT MATTERS MOST

What matters most in losing fat from your waistline are the following practices:

• The overall consumption of calories must be lower than your energy expenditure on a daily basis.

• Superhydration, the continual sipping of at least 1 gallon of ice-cold water a day, accelerates fat loss and stomach flattening.

• Hard, brief strength training ensures that the resulting weight loss is from fat. Strength training also improves the shape, firmness, and contours of the midsection muscles.

It's time, once again, to get serious about this three-pronged formula.

THE EATING PLAN

The eating plan here is a combination of the most popular food selections from chapter 20 and chapter 21. Men will adhere to 1,435 calories a day and the women to 1,255 calories per day, distributed over six small meals. The amount of calories stays the same throughout the six-week program. The midmorning, midafternoon, and late-night snacks are Champion Nutrition products (see www.Champion-Nutrition.com). If these are unavailable, you may substitute similar shake mixes and energy bars. Just make sure the calorie counts are the same.

MENUS FOR WEEKS 1–6

BREAKFAST = 320 CALORIES

1 bagel (Lender's New York Style, plain or blueberry), frozen, toasted (250)

1 slice Swiss processed cheese (70)

Noncaloric beverage

MIDMORNING SNACK

Men = 140 calories

Women = 95 calories

Men: ½ Champion Ultramet packet mixed with 7 ounces of cold water (140)

Women: ½ Champion Ultramet Lite packet mixed with 6 ounces of cold water (95)

LUNCH = 300 CALORIES

SANDWICH

2 slices whole-wheat bread (140)

3 ounces white meat chicken or turkey (120)

2 teaspoons Hellmann's Light Mayonnaise (33)

2 tomato slices (14)

Noncaloric beverage

MIDAFTERNOON SNACK

Men = 140 calories

Women = 95 calories

Men: ½ Champion Ultramet packet mixed with 7 ounces of cold water (140)

Women: ½ Champion Ultramet Lite packet mixed with 6 ounces of cold water (95)

DINNER = 300 CALORIES

Choice of tuna salad or one of three frozen microwave meals and a noncaloric beverage:

TUNA SALAD DINNER (300)

In a large bowl, mix the following ingredients:

½ 6-ounce can chunk light tuna in water, drained (75)

½ cup (4 ounces) whole kernel corn, canned, no salt added (60)

¼ cup (2 ounces) dark red kidney beans, canned (65)

½ apple, chopped (50)

1 tablespoon Hellmann's Light, Reduced-Calorie Mayonnaise (50)

1 tablespoon sweet pickle relish (20)

FROZEN MICROWAVE DINNERS

BLACKENED CHICKEN, HEALTHY CHOICE (320)

SANTA FE–STYLE RICE AND BEANS, LEAN CUISINE EVERYDAY FAVORITES (300)

LASAGNA WITH MEAT SAUCE, MICHELINA'S AUTHENTICO (290)

LATE-NIGHT SNACK

Men = 180 calories

Women = 90 calories

Men: 1 Champion SnacBar (180)

Women: ½ Champion SnacBar (90)

Notes: Noncaloric beverages are any type of water, soft drink, tea, or coffee with zero calories and no caffeine. For whole-wheat bread, try to select one that lists as the first ingredient whole, sprouted, or cracked grain.

SUPERHYDRATION

Flip back to chapter 19, page 177, to review and apply the superhydration schedule for weeks 1–6. Start by consuming 1 gallon of ice-cold water each day for week 1. Gradually work up to $1\frac{5}{8}$ gallons, or 208 ounces, per day during week 6. The cold water will keep you moving and grooving throughout the day and night. Remember, plenty of chilled water is necessary to synergize your eating and exercising.

ABDOMINAL FOCUS BOWFLEX ROUTINES

Here are the Bowflex routines I recommend for the Abdominal Focus course. You will add two new exercises after each two-week segment. Perform one set of 8 to 12 repetitions in all exercises, with one exception. During weeks 5 and 6, you will include the Stomach Vacuum, which is not really an exercise but more of a trick that I'll describe later. Practice the appropriate routine three nonconsecutive days per week.

WEEKS 1 AND 2

1. Seated Abdominal Crunch

2. Leg Curl

3. Leg Extension

4. Lying Shoulder Pullover

5. Bench Press

6. Seated Oblique Crunch

If you are unsure how to perform any of these exercises, complete descriptions and photographs are found in chapters 6, 7, and 8.

Each routine begins and ends with an abdominal exercise—a good way to emphasize a specific body part. The Seated Abdominal Crunch and the Seated Oblique Crunch are both short-range movements. As a result, it's especially important that you move very deliberately as you slowly contract your midsection muscles. Be sure to keep your abdominals tight throughout the entire set. Do not rest between repetitions.

WEEKS 3 AND 4

1. Seated Abdominal Crunch

2. Leg Curl

3. Leg Extension

4. Lying Shoulder Pullover

5. Reverse Grip Pulldown*

6. Bench Press

7. Seated Oblique Crunch

8. Side Bend with Body Weight*

*New exercise

During Weeks 3 and 4, you'll add the Reverse Grip Pulldown and the Side Bend with Body Weight. A description of the Reverse Grip Pulldown is on page 66. The Side Bend is a productive freehand exercise that does not require a Bowflex machine. It targets the external and internal oblique muscles on the sides of your waist. Here's how to do it:

Side Bend: Stand with your feet hip-width apart. Extend your arms above your head and interlace your fingers. Stand tall and reach toward the ceiling. When you achieve maximum height, start bending laterally to the left. Pause briefly in the stretched position and reach again with your hands, this time maximally to the left. Return slowly to the top center position. Do not let your arms move forward. Keep them extended and directly over the top of your head. Reach toward the ceiling with both hands and repeat bending to the left for eight repetitions. Rest for a few seconds with your hands hanging at your sides. Perform the movement to your right side in a similar manner for the same number of repetitions.

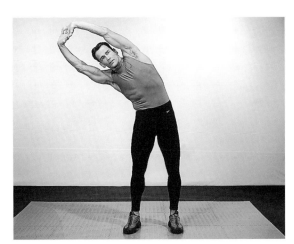

Side Bend: Reach and bend laterally, first to one side for the required repetitions, then to the other side.

WEEKS 5 AND 6

1. Seated Abdominal Crunch

2. Leg Curl

3. Leg Extension

4. Leg Press*

5. Lying Shoulder Pullover

6. Reverse Grip Pulldown

7. Bench Press

8. Seated Oblique Crunch

9. Side Bend

10. Stomach Vacuum*

*New exercise

I've added the Leg Press for this segment and the Stomach Vacuum, a trick I learned years ago from a champion bodybuilder who used it during his onstage posing routine, where it always caused the audience to go wild with amazement. What he would do was suck in his stomach to such a degree that you could almost see his backbone from the front. He was able to do this because he had unusual control over his transversus abdominis muscle, which is a wide, paper-thin muscle that stretches horizontally beneath the better-known rectus abdominis muscle. I want you to practice the Stomach Vacuum as your final exercise during weeks 5 and 6.

Stomach Vacuum: Lie on your back on the floor, or on the flat bench of the Bowflex machine. Make sure your stomach is relatively empty. Place your hands across the bottom of your rib cage and top of your abdominals. Take a normal breath and forcibly blow out as much air as possible. This should require about ten seconds. Now here's the challenging part: Suck in your stomach to the maximum degree— while not taking in any air during the process. The transversus abdominis muscle has to be called into action for this to occur. If you're doing it properly, you'll feel a concave formation under your rib cage.

You won't be able to hold the vacuum formation very long. Try the vacuum several times while lying down. If you feel a little light-headed, that's normal. Rest a bit longer between repetitions.

Stand now and try the vacuum in front of a mirror. Remove your shirt so you can see what's happening. At first, the vacuum is more difficult to do standing than lying, but with a little practice you should be able to master it in a standing position.

Perform the Stomach Vacuum for four repetitions at the end of your Bowflex routine during weeks 5 and 6. After two weeks of practice, your transversus abdominis muscle should be much stronger. And you should be able to suck in your stomach to a much greater degree. Keep practicing and you'll get better and better.

REALITY RULES!

For the past ten years, most fitness-minded people in the United States seem to have been obsessed with muscular midsections and great abdominals. Being realistic in your goals and your expectations, however, leads to a much healthier attitude. Not everyone has the genetics to have abdominals like Peter Fleck. But we all can improve, we all can get better. If—after going through the Abdominal Focus course—you're still disappointed with your midsection, then you probably still have more fat to lose. The solution is simply to go through the entire six-week course again.

Brad Knuth, who was part of the group that included Peter Fleck, went through the six-week plan four times before he was "reasonably satisfied" with his midsection. In reality, Knuth—after losing almost 50 pounds of fat and 8 inches off his waist—would probably have to remain committed to the program for another six months before he could become "completely satisfied." And even then, he would not have the rippling abdominals of Peter Fleck.

Reality can be a harsh friend that consistently keeps you aware of the value of hard work, science, and meaning in life. Be glad that losing fat, building muscle, and getting a lean waistline require hard work and attention to science. Once you get what you want, you'll be less likely to part with it.

That's reality.

Reality rules!

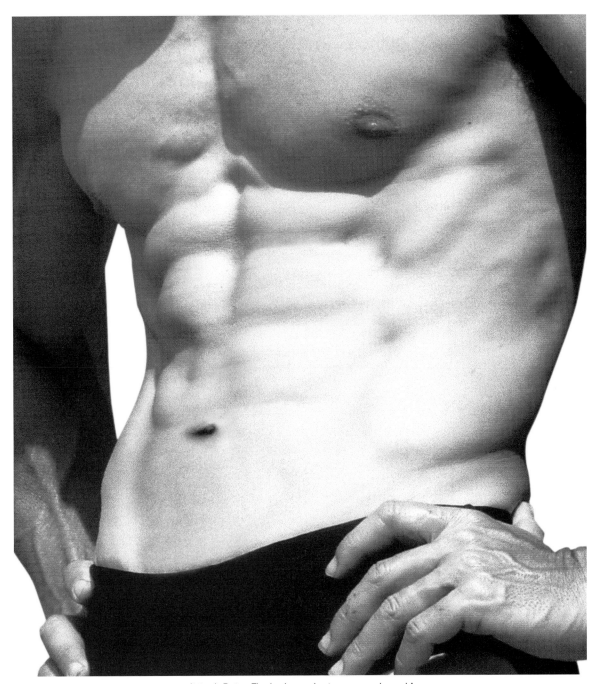

It took Peter Fleck six weeks to earn a six-pack!

24

A THICKER CHEST:

A TWO-WEEK BLITZ
FOR PUMPED PECTORALS

MEN, WOULD YOU BE WILLING TO TRY a new Bowflex routine if I told you it would add size to your pectoral muscles and thicken your entire chest in only two weeks?

Well, I have a special blitz that, if performed correctly, will do just that. It will pump you up in record time, I promise. The secret to my pump-you-up-in-record-time promise involves two parts. One, the chest portion of the Bowflex routine, uses pre-exhaustion. That's where you don't rest between back-to-back performances of two related exercises. Two, I recommend that you add creatine, a dietary supplement, to your daily superhydration schedule, along with the right amount of sugar. The resulting creatine-sugar drink helps pull fluids into your working muscles, both during and after the routine. The entire process, you might say, boosts the blitz.

Here's a look at the Bowflex routine, with appropriate descriptions of the exercises.

(*Warning:* This two-week blitz is *not* for beginners. It's for advanced trainees only. Do not try this routine unless you've trained on Bowflex for at least six months.)

BOWFLEX ROUTINE: THICKER-CHEST BLITZ

1. Chest Fly, immediately followed by
2. Bench Press
3. Incline Chest Fly, immediately followed by
4. Decline Bench Press

Bonus exercise: Negative Push-Up

5. Leg Extension/Leg Curl
6. Leg Press
7. Standing Lateral Raise
8. Lying Shoulder Pullover
9. Standing Biceps Curl
10. Seated Abdominal Crunch

DESCRIPTION OF PRE-EXHAUSTION EXERCISES

Chest Fly. Remember to place the pulleys in the wide position, if applicable to your machine, on all chest exercises. Adjust the bench to a 45-degree incline and grasp a handle in each hand. Your job on the Chest Fly is to isolate the pectoralis major muscles without requiring much of the triceps. Straighten your arms directly over your chest. Now bend your elbows slightly, approximately 10 degrees, and keep them at this angle throughout the movement. This is the top, the starting position, with your hands almost touching.

Move the handles outward and downward into a comfortable stretch, which you should feel across your chest. Pull, do not push, the handles back to the starting position. Remember, the idea is to involve your pectoral muscles, not your triceps, so keep that slight bend in your elbows.

Do between 8 and 12 repetitions in good form. On your last repetition, without even a pause, immediately go into the Bench Press.

Bench Press. Now, you're going to use those triceps, which you've been saving, to force your pre-exhausted pectorals to a deeper level of fatigue. With the handles straight over your chest, bend your elbows and bring your hands near your shoulders. Press the handles smoothly back to the starting position. Repeat for at least 8 repetitions, which may be tough to do. Even if you can't quite get 8, don't give up. Keep pushing in good form, and breathing, for at least 5 seconds. Maybe you will succeed.

After that final effort, carefully get out of the machine, roll your shoulders and move your arms some, and get ready for the Incline Chest Fly.

Incline Chest Fly. Compared to the Chest Fly and the Bench Press, you'll need to lighten the Power Rods by approximately 20 percent on the Incline

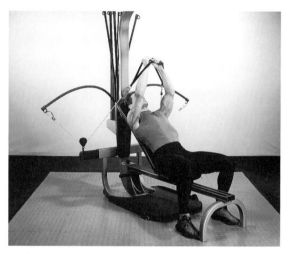

Incline Chest Fly: Keep a slight bend in your elbows as you lower the handles for a moderate stretch of your pectoral muscles. Pull the handles back to the over-shoulder position and repeat.

Chest Fly. The performance of this exercise is similar to the Chest Fly, except your arms are higher in relationship to your torso. A higher-arm position involves more of the pectoralis major muscles near your collarbones.

Begin by grasping the handles from the seated, 45-degree bench position, and then straightening your arms over your chest. But instead of keeping your arms perpendicular to your torso, incline them 20 to 30 degrees higher. The handles should now be over your neck, rather than over your chest. Bend your elbows slightly and keep them bent throughout the movement.

Move the handles outward and downward for a controlled stretch. Smoothly make the transition from lowering to raising and pull the handles back to the over-neck position. Repeat for 8 to 12 repetitions. After the final repetition, lower the handles to your shoulders and get ready for the Decline Bench Press.

Decline Bench Press. This is a terrific chest exercise, especially when it's performed immediately after the Incline Chest Fly. What you're doing is going from an upper-chest emphasis to a lower-chest emphasis, which is the area hit by the Decline Bench Press. In the Decline Bench Press, you push the handles more toward your knees, as opposed to over your chest.

Start by straightening your arms over your chest,

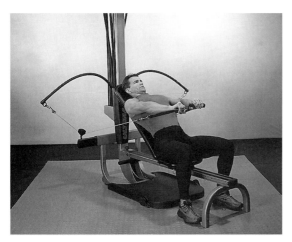

Decline Bench Press: Flex your elbows and guide the handles to the sides of your rib cage. Stretch and repeat the decline pressing for maximum repetitions.

then decline them 20 to 30 degrees. The farther down your arms go, the more you involve your triceps, which is good. You're going to need as much triceps involvement as you can muster to get at those deeper pectoral muscles.

Bend your elbows and let the handles return near your shoulders. Continue the decline pressing for 8 or more repetitions. As before, 8 repetitions are probably going to be a real bear to complete. Stay focused and finish the set. After several workouts, and as you get the hang of what's going on, you should be able to do 12 repetitions. When you can successfully do 12 repetitions of the Decline Bench Press, then I want you to progress to the bonus exercise, which is what I call a Negative Push-Up. The bonus exercise is important to the overall effect.

Negative Push-Up. You won't need your Bowflex machine for this exercise. All you need is your body's weight and a floor to lie on facedown. After the final repetition of the Decline Bench Press, move off the machine and get on the floor as fast as you can in the top position of a standard push-up. In other words, you're on your toes and hands with your arms straight and your body stiff. Your job is to concentrate on the lowering, or negative, portion of this exercise.

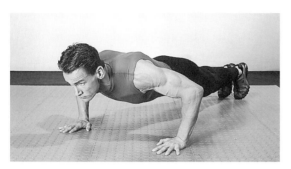

Negative Push-Up: Halfway down, at the count of 5, the tough part of this movement is just beginning. Keep descending, ever so slowly, until your chest touches the floor. Repeat this lowering-only exercise for three or more repetitions.

Lower your body to the floor by bending your arms as you count to 10 slowly. You should be halfway down in 5 seconds and almost all the way down in 8 or 9 seconds. Touch the floor with your chest at the 10-second mark. Do not push yourself up to the top position. Use your legs to get up. Place your knees on the floor, raise your chest, straighten your arms, and slide back on your toes. Repeat the Negative Push-Up for at least 3 repetitions, which sounds easy until you actually try it—following those other four chest exercises. Try to add another repetition with each workout.

OTHER EXERCISES IN THE ROUTINE

The remaining six exercises are performed in a normal manner. If you are unsure about how to do any of them, please turn back to the descriptions and illustrations in chapters 6, 7, and 8. You'll notice that the Leg Extension/Leg Curl comes after the chest exercises. This means that the Leg Extension is alternated with the Leg Curl. Do not do them both during the same exercise session. Alternate between them.

THE CREATINE SPLASH

From chapter 15, you learned that most of the current dietary supplements that are classified as ergogenic aids are little more than expensive placebos. Creatine, however, is an ergogenic aid that actually does some of what it claims to do. Properly consumed, creatine can contribute to muscular size and strength.

Creatine is a proteinlike substance manufactured naturally by your body and stored in your muscles. Studies show that in your body, creatine acts similar to the way cylinders operate in an automobile engine. Absorbing it in large amounts is like boosting the number of cylinders in your muscles.

Interestingly, creatine is also found in beef, pork, and fish. So why can't you get more creatine simply by eating more meat? Well, you can—if you like your meat raw and eat several pounds of it a day. Cooking destroys much of the creatine in meat.

That's why in the early 1990s researchers began experimenting with combining certain amino acids with other chemicals in the laboratory to produce a rich source of creatine called creatine monohydrate. Creatine monohydrate, which is a white powder, can be mixed with water and consumed several times a day to get a larger-than-average amount in the muscles to achieve a loaded effect.

I personally tried creatine loading several times on my own body in 1993 with good results. Furthermore, I experimented with it in a number of bodybuilding studies in 1994 and 1995 with even better results.

It didn't take long for supplement companies to get involved in a major way. In 2000, creatine products registered more than $100 million in sales.

Today, at your local nutrition store, you'll find liquid creatine, creatine with dextrose, low-carbohydrate creatine, creatine candy chews, effervescent creatine, and micronized creatine, as well as plain creatine monohydrate. I've given most of them a try, but I've never had better results than with the formula I designed in 1994, with the help of a University of Florida chemistry student.

The formula requires some time and effort, and it's kind of messy, but it does a remarkable job of loading and packing creatine into your muscle cells. You'll feel the effects in as little as three days. Here's the thinking behind the formula.

MY CREATINE FORMULA

In 1994 I found that the loading of creatine monohydrate could be improved in two ways. First, apply superhydration to creatine. In other words, dissolve the daily dosage of creatine in a gallon of water and sip it continuously throughout the day. Second, add common sugar to the solution. Sugar elevates insulin levels and insulin facilitates creatine absorption into the muscles.

Here are the procedures that I've used in helping bodybuilders add mass to their working muscles. I recommend that you apply them, according to the directions, as a part of the Thicker-Chest Blitz.

CREATINE-LOADING PROCEDURES

The entire process will be easier if you have these items:

1 large thermos jug, 2-gallon capacity

1 32-ounce plastic bottle with straw

1 digital, battery-operated food scale

1 large wooden spoon

1 5-pound bag of granulated white sugar

1 large bottle (210 grams) creatine
  monohydrate dietary supplement

12 ice cubes

Do the following before you begin your day:

1. Place 1 gallon of water into a large thermos jug.

2. Spoon out 20 grams of creatine monohydrate (1 heaping teaspoon equals approximately 5 grams, but calculate the precise weight on a digital food scale).

3. Pour 20 grams of creatine into your water. Stir gently with the large wooden spoon for 15 seconds or until it is dissolved.

4. Weigh out 104 grams of sugar (approximately ½ cup), which has the energy value of 400 calories.

5. Empty the sugar into the creatine solution and stir vigorously for 1 minute or until the sugar is dissolved.

6. Add ice cubes to the thermos to chill the solution. Your objective is to drink over the next fourteen hours at least 1 gallon of the creatine-sugar solution. The thermos allows you to carry the mixture with you wherever you go.

7. Draw into your 32-ounce plastic bottle an initial quart of solution and sip from it over the next several hours. Most people find they can consume the fluid easier through a straw than they can by drinking it from a glass. Having the solution cold also helps.

8. Keep refilling your 32-ounce bottle and sipping until the thermos is depleted. Try to spread the 128 ounces or more evenly over twelve to fourteen hours.

9. Wash the thermos and plastic bottle with hot soapy water at the end of the day.

10. Repeat the same directions daily for seven days.

11. Stop loading after the first week and move to a maintenance dosage for the second week. For a maintenance dosage, take 5 grams of creatine monohydrate mixed in 4 ounces of water each morning after breakfast. Continue with the daily superhydration by drinking 1 gallon of cold water.

Note: Caffeine cancels some of the loading effects of creatine. Do not consume caffeinated drinks such as coffee, tea, or certain sodas during the loading phase.

USING THE TWO-WEEK BLITZ

Do the Thicker-Chest Blitz on your Bowflex machine three times per week for two consecutive weeks only. Continuing with such an intense, pre-exhaustion routine for longer than two weeks would soon lead to overtraining. Return to your normal workouts for at least three months. Then, if your chest still needs additional specialization, you can try the Thicker-Chest Blitz again.

Do the creatine loading for only one week simultaneous to the first week of the Thicker-Chest Blitz. Use the maintenance solution of creatine during the second week. You can continue with the maintenance solution of creatine for an additional thirty days, if you like.

Of course, during the two-week blitz, you don't want to skimp on your calories. Make sure you have three or four nutritious meals plus a couple of snacks each day. Extra rest and sleep will also help the muscle-building process.

PUMPED TO GROW

Now, it's up to you. Bend the bow and sip the creatine until your pectorals are pumped to the max.

Blitz. Rest. Recover. Blitz. Rest. Recover. And grow!

It's just that simple.

25
ACCENT ON ARMS:

A TWO-WEEK BLITZ
FOR BIGGER BICEPS AND TRICEPS

WAS THERE EVER A FITNESS-MINDED man who didn't want bigger biceps and triceps? I doubt it. This is still the most popular subject in any magazine concerned with male muscular development.

Here's a two-week blitz that involves the performance of several unusual exercises on your Bowflex machine. Once you've completed the routine for the first time, I assure you that your biceps and triceps will burn, pump, and ache like nothing you've ever experienced. Do this properly, three times per week, for two consecutive weeks—combined with a little extra rest and sleep, nutritious meals, and the creatine-sugar-superhydration schedule from chapter 24—and you've got my personal guarantee that you'll be rewarded with measurable increases in the circumference of your upper arms.

(*Warning:* This two-week blitz is *not* for beginners. It's for advanced trainees only. Do not try this routine unless you've trained on a Bowflex machine for at least six months.)

BOWFLEX ROUTINE: BIGGER-ARMS BLITZ

1. Seated Triceps Extension, Negative Emphasized

2. Seated Biceps Curl, Negative Emphasized

3. Leg Curl

4. Leg Extension

5. Seated Calf Raise

6. Reverse Grip Pulldown

7. Shoulder Shrug

8. Seated Biceps Curl, Negative Emphasized

9. Seated Triceps Extension, Negative Emphasized

Bonus exercise: Negative Push-Up

Note: Perform the bracketed exercises with minimal rest in between.

NEGATIVE EMPHASIZED

"Negative emphasized" in the context of this discussion means to do the positive (pushing) part of the exercise in an easier, faster-than-normal way, and the negative (lowering) portion in a harder, slower-than-normal manner. You'll understand what I'm referring to on the first Bowflex exercise.

Seated Triceps Extension, Negative Emphasized. Done in good form, with your upper arms fixed, a seated extension does a great job at isolating your triceps. But it's difficult to do this exercise in good form because your upper arms and elbows tend to move, which brings into action other muscles to assist the triceps. In reality, what most trainees end up doing on this exercise is sort of a combination bench press and triceps extension, which is not good. Watching several people perform the exercise in this manner, however, prompted me to experiment with the movement. Soon, I had an improved way of doing it, which I called negative emphasized.

In the normal seated position, with the handles near your shoulders, bench press them over your chest. Raise the handles higher as if you're completing an Incline Bench Press and move the handles together until your thumbs touch. Stabilize your upper arms and slowly lower the handles to your eyebrows in 10 seconds. That's right—slowly count to 10 during the lowering, or negative. Once you reach your eyebrows, smoothly drop your elbows and hands down to the bench press position and quickly push the handles overhead. Raise and reposition the handles, take a deep breath, and lower for another 10-second repetition.

What you're doing here is a fast, positive bench press, which takes about 2 seconds, and a slow, negative triceps extension, which takes about 10 seconds. After 5 or 6 repetitions, your bench press will become slower and your triceps extension will be-

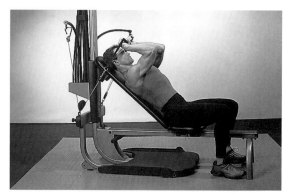

Seated Triceps Extension, Negative Emphasized: Take 10 seconds to lower the handles slowly to your eyebrows.

come faster. When you can no longer control the lowering speed, stop the exercise.

If you've selected the resistance on the Power Rods correctly, you should be able to do 8 slow, negative-emphasized repetitions. When you can do 12, add 5 pounds of the Power Rods to each side.

Seated Biceps Curl, Negative Emphasized. You're going to do something similar with your biceps. From the same seated, 45-degree position, curl the handles to your shoulders. That should be fairly easy, even with a heavy resistance because in a seated position, the range is short and the Power Rods don't bend very much. Remember in chapter 5, when I noted that the best Bowflex exercises require a complete bend of the bows? Well, the Seated Biceps Curl is not normally one of my recommended exercises because of this.

To improve the range of movement on some

seated exercises, simply stand up. Standing up lengthens the movement and allows more bending to occur in the Power Rods. But you can accomplish the same thing from a seated position if you lean your upper body forward, increasing the distance and adding to the bending of the bows. Then, from the leaning-forward position, while holding the handles near your shoulders and your biceps fully contracted, do the negative, lowering phase of the movement very slowly during a count of 10.

After the negative phase, sit back and curl the handles quickly to your shoulders in one fluid move, lean forward, and do another negative-emphasized repetition. You'll involve your biceps more if you remember to keep your upper arms stable as you uncurl the handles. Also, keep your knees close together in the leaning-forward position so the handles can pass easily by your thighs.

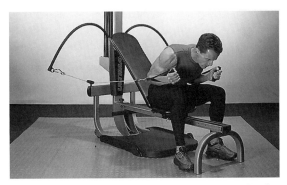

Keep your elbows flexed as you lean forward. Leaning forward improves the resistance on the Power Rods and makes the exercise more effective.

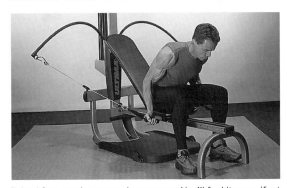

Take 10 seconds to uncurl your arms. You'll feel it more if, at the halfway point, you try to touch your knuckles to the floor.

Specifically, what you're doing on the Seated Biceps Curl is cheating on the positive phase by shortening the movement and then using your abdominals and hip flexors to lengthen the distance to perform a maximum-bend-in-the-bows, heavy-resistance, negative-emphasized repetition.

Once again, you should strive for 8 to 12 negative repetitions in this exercise. Start out doing as many 10-second lowering repetitions as you

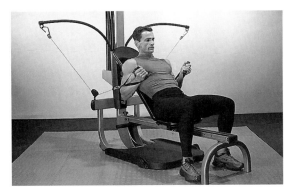

Curl the handles quickly to your shoulders.

can before you have to go a little faster, which won't take long, especially if you get the hang of moving quickly back to the leaning-forward starting position. This is an intense exercise, so be sure and keep your neck and face relaxed as you breathe. Stop when you can no longer control the lowering.

REPEAT AGAIN,
BUT REVERSE THE ORDER

Perform a second set of the Triceps Extension and the Biceps Curl at the end of the routine. But for these sets, reverse the order—do the Biceps Curl before the Triceps Extension.

The reason for this is that during the second week you will finish off your routine with the same Negative Push-Up I described on page 231. The Negative Push-Up was used in chapter 24 to add a final pump to the pectorals. It's applied in this chapter, however, as a finisher for the triceps.

After the final repetition of the Seated Triceps Extension, immediately get out of the machine, down on the floor, and into the top position of a push-up. Your goal is do a 10-second, lowering-only repetition, and repeat it five or six times. Stop the Negative Push-Up when you can no longer control the lowering.

OTHER EXERCISES

Five other exercises, which cover your lower body and torso, make up the rest of this routine. If needed, refer to their descriptions in chapters 6, 7, and 8.

USING THE BIGGER-ARMS BLITZ

Do the Bigger-Arms Blitz routine three times per week for two consecutive weeks. Do not perform it more often than three times per week and don't do it for longer than two weeks. More is not better when it comes to amount of exercise. Harder is better.

In fact, some very strong Bowflex trainees might have better results from applying the Bigger-Arms Blitz only twice a week. If you think you might fall into that advanced category, go with twice a week.

After the Bigger-Arms Blitz, return to your normal workouts for at least three months. You can repeat the blitz after that.

CREATINE-SUPERHYDRATION

For maximum effect, I'd suggest that you employ the creatine-sugar-superhydration schedule from page 233. Creatine loading will help to add volume to your biceps and triceps. And don't forget about getting extra rest and sleep, as well as plenty of nutritious calories for the entire two-week blitz.

MAXIMIZING MUSCULAR SIZE

An important factor in building bigger biceps and triceps in the blitz is your ability to move efficiently between exercises 1 and 2, and exercises 8 and 9. On the Bowflex machine, if the Power Rods are selected carefully, you do *not* have to drop the handles, get out of the machine, readjust the resistance, get back into the machine, and grasp the handles again. If your hands start to tire from holding the handles, then you're probably gripping them too tightly. There must be little rest between the two exercises. A 4- or 5-second pause between them can cut your size gains in half. If you absolutely have to change the Power Rods, then get a training partner to do it for you.

In fact, I recommend that all people who go through the arm or the chest blitz team up with a partner. Your partner can talk you through each repetition of each exercise, count your 10-second negatives, record accurately your performance with a pencil on your workout chart, and motivate you consistently during those important last repetitions.

A good training partner should also be a stickler for good form, as you should be when you train him or her. As you should know by now, there are a lot of little things that, when caught and corrected, will make your Bowflex workouts harder and more productive.

BIGGER BICEPS
AND TRICEPS *NOW!*

Your upper arms will most definitely become bigger and stronger not in a matter of months but in two weeks. The Bigger-Arms Blitz works, but only if you're willing to put forth the intensity and attention to detail.

Commit now and make it happen.

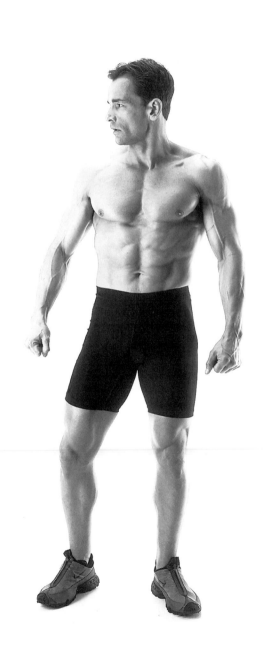

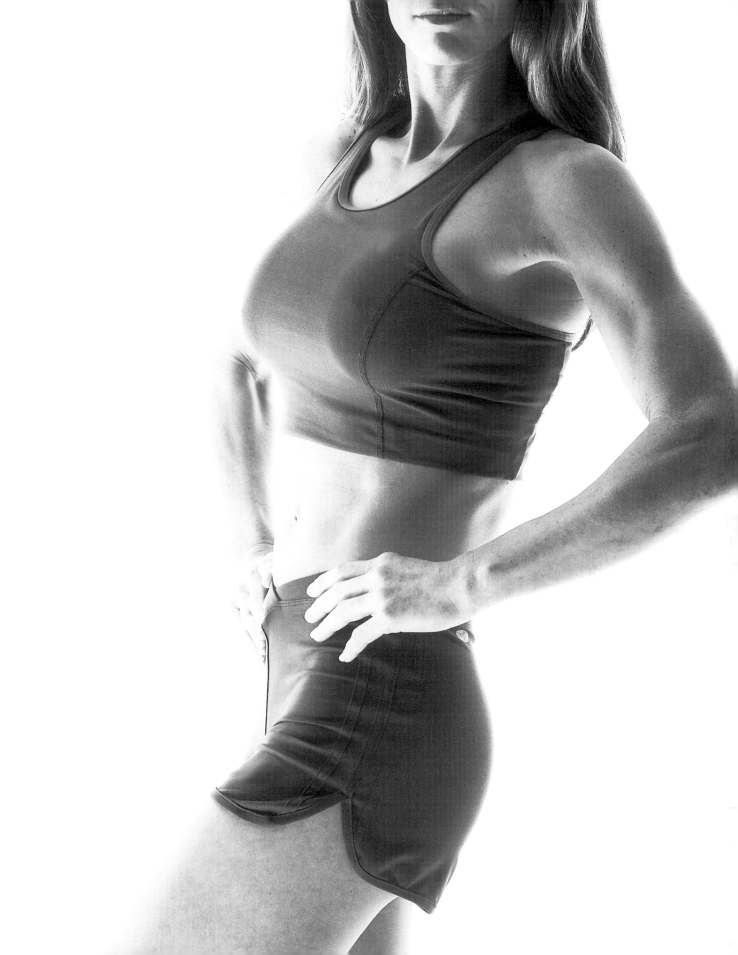

26

THOSE LAST 5 POUNDS:

30 TIPS ON HOW TO LOSE THEM

IN THE QUEST TO REACH YOUR body-leanness goal, those last 5 pounds always seem to be the hardest to lose. Here are 30 tips that will help you reach your goal more efficiently.

These tips provide a review of many of the guidelines that you've already been practicing, and they also serve as a primer for long-term maintenance.

• Lose fat for yourself—not for your spouse or friends.

• Set realistic goals. Progress one day at a time, and be patient.

• Learn to say, "No thank you," when people offer you food.

• Hold a conference and explain your fat-loss program to family, friends, and coworkers. They are more likely to be understanding and supportive of your goals then.

• Pace your eating by putting your fork down between bites. The more slowly you eat, the more quickly you'll feel full.

• Don't use place settings with intense colors such as warm red, bright yellow, lime green, or orange. These colors tend to stimulate the appetite. Food offered on white or pastel plates is less appealing to hearty eaters.

• Go grocery shopping only on a full stomach.

• Shop from a written list of necessities. Walking through the supermarket unprepared can be hazardous to your leanness.

• Don't skip meals. You'll only overeat later.

• Eat smaller meals more frequently. Doing so keeps your blood-sugar level at an even keel, controls your appetite, and facilitates fat loss.

• Learn to distinguish appetite from true hunger. When the urge to eat hits, wait several minutes to see if it passes.

• Combat the candy habit. Instead of eating a piece of candy, brush your teeth. The tingling of the toothpaste may make your craving go away.

• Bring your lunch to work whenever possible. You have more control when you prepare your own food.

• Diet with a friend. Many successful fat-loss programs rely heavily on group support. Start your own, even with just one other person.

• Superhydrate daily to promote greater fat loss and muscle building.

• Remain uncomfortably cool throughout the day to allow your skin's heating mechanism to adjust to a lower level.

• Cut back on evening TV. Studies show that people who watch a lot of TV tend to be overfat. Heavier people agree that TV encourages them not only to sit but to snack.

• Suck on a lemon or lime if you feel you're about to binge.

• Keep plenty of crunchy foods such as raw vegetables and air-popped popcorn on hand for emergencies. They're high in fiber and filling.

• Freeze fresh fruit such as grapes, blueberries, or strawberries. They'll take longer to eat and you'll be satisfied with less.

• Sip hot soup. A bowl of low-calorie soup can be wonderfully filling.

• Substitute plain yogurt for mayonnaise and sour cream in dips and dressings and on baked potatoes.

• Avoid boredom. There is probably no bigger diet buster. Too often, time on your hands translates to food in your mouth. Keep busy.

• Walk moderately after your evening meal. You'll temporarily burn more calories.

• Chew sugarless gum for oral gratification. You may find it helpful in ending a meal, too.

• Give away the "fat clothes" in your closet. Keeping larger sizes around undermines your confidence in being able to maintain your fat loss.

• Sit straight and stand tall. Proper posture burns more calories than slouching, in addition to making your belly look smaller.

• Turn down the volume. Your stereo could be fattening because loud noise produces stress chemicals that may make people overeat.

• Don't let your muscles shrink and your fat expand as you age. Build up muscle to elevate your metabolism, improve your shape, and burn more calories. A pound of muscle requires 37.5 calories a day; a pound of fat uses only 2.

• Exercise harder, briefer, and smarter on Bowflex to significantly increase your muscle size and strength.

27
MORE PROGRESS:
A FEW TWISTS FOR CONTINUED SUCCESS

IF YOU RECENTLY COMPLETED ONE of the six-week fat-loss courses in Part IV, then it's time for you to weigh yourself and measure your body fat and your body parts in the same way you did in chapter 19. You might want to pose for some "after" photographs as well. Once you've finished, you'll want to do a few calculations and compare your results with some of my group averages.

POUNDS AND INCHES LOST

I've worked with thousands of men and women over the past twenty years in various fat-loss projects that involved reduced-calorie dieting, superhydration, and strength training. From these studies, I've deduced the following six-week averages:

SIX-WEEK AVERAGES (IN POUNDS)

	Men	Women
Weight Lost	17.750	10.375
Muscle Gained	3.750	3.000
Fat Lost	21.500	13.375

SIX-WEEK AVERAGES, INCHES LOST

	Men	Women
Waist	3.250	2.750
Hips	1.750	1.875
Thighs	3.125	3.375

My typical participant was in his or her mid-thirties. The average man was 5 feet 11 inches tall and weighed approximately 210 pounds. The average woman was 5 feet 4 inches tall and weighed approximately 160 pounds.

If your age, height, and weight are within 10 percent of my average participant, then you could reasonably expect to see similar losses in pounds and inches. Don't be alarmed if your before-and-after differences are less than average. They can be 20 percent lower and still fall within the normal range. If you see above-average results, congratulations. You should be elated.

Since we're talking about averages, there are several variables to consider in making valid comparisons. For example, I've found that participants younger than age thirty achieve better-than-average results while those over age fifty get slightly less-than-average results. Height is a major factor too. Taller individuals do significantly better than shorter people.

Finally, simple division shows that the average man can expect to lose 0.512 pound each day and 3.58 pounds each week. The average woman can expect to lose 0.318 pound each day and 2.226 pounds each week.

If you've accurately measured your body weight and body fat percentage before and after your completion of any of the six-week plans, your improvements should be near these numbers and you should feel proud of these results.

MUSCLE ADDED

Bowflex builds muscle. There's no doubt about it. I've seen it happen in participant after participant after participant. You should be able to verify the amount of muscle you've built while measuring your body fat. Simply subtract your weight loss from your fat loss. If you've performed the calculations correctly, your fat loss should be more than your weight loss. The difference is the amount of muscle you've gained.

Most men I've worked with, and these are men who have *not* been previously involved in strength training, add an average of 3.75 pounds of muscle on their bodies in six weeks. That's 0.625 pound of muscle per week. Women build slightly less: 3 pounds in six weeks or 0.5 pound per week.

If you don't have access to skin fold calipers, then you can estimate your muscle gain by examining closely your workout records. Most men and women,

if they are progressing 1 repetition per exercise per workout, get approximately 5-percent stronger each week on each exercise. A 5-percent improvement in strength in each exercise for one week equals approximately 0.5 pound of muscle gain. A 30-percent strength improvement in six weeks, therefore, equals 3 pounds of muscle.

Compare the resistance you supplied on the Power Rods for 10 repetitions of an exercise during your first or second workout with the resistance you used on your last workout for 10 repetitions. Don't be surprised if you are 30-percent to 40-percent stronger. A stronger muscle is a larger muscle and a larger muscle is a stronger muscle.

Do the calculations. Gaining 3 to 4 pounds of muscle is a possibility, and it's probably noticeable in your photographs.

FULL-BODY PHOTOGRAPHS

If you took full-body photographs of yourself in a bathing suit six weeks ago, you'll want to take them again. You should see dramatic improvement when you compare your before and after pictures side by side. Make sure the setup in both sets of pictures is exactly the same.

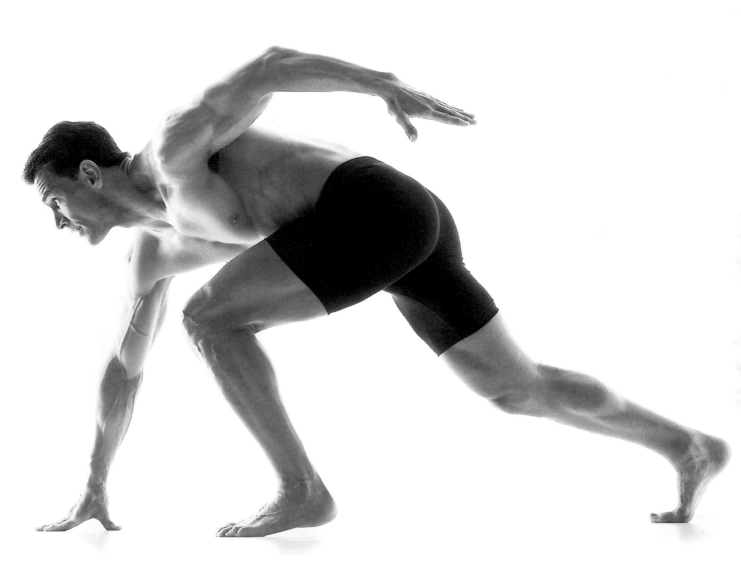

He Surpassed His Goal

Richard L. Clelland, age sixty-five, is retired and lives in East Peoria, Illinois. He's been married for forty-five years and has two children. He bought a Bowflex Power Pro in June of 2000 because he wanted to lose weight. Also, at 5 feet 9 inches and 240 pounds, he suffered from chronic low-back pain. "I knew I had to do something about my health," Richard noted, "and Bowflex offered me hope."

Richard was motivated by the Body-Leanness Plan. He applied the eating recommendations, the superhydration schedule, and the twenty-minute workout for an entire year.

"Steady is the way I'd describe my progress," Richard remembered. "I dropped about 5 pounds each month. You know that back pain I had? At the end of six months it disappeared. That certainly added to my motivation."

At the end of twelve months, Richard was 66 pounds lighter and had reduced the size of his waist by 10 inches.

"When I started the Bowflex program," Richard said, "I wanted to lose 60 pounds. I actually surpassed my goal by 6 pounds.

"My friends, at first, could not believe my weight loss. Now that I've achieved what I set out to do—and maintained my weight loss for more than a year—they want to buy my Bowflex. *No way.*

"Without it, I'd probably balloon up to 240 pounds again."

WHAT TO DO NEXT

Approximately 50 percent of the people I work with reach their fat-loss goals in six weeks. If you're one of these people, then chapter 28 discusses a maintenance plan that will help you keep off the fat.

The other 50 percent of my participants still want to get rid of more pounds and inches. They may have reached their goal, but they still want to continue. If you're in either of these categories, here's what to do.

COMMIT AGAIN

Decide now to commit for another six weeks. But don't expect the exact results as before. With the same level of compliance, you'll get approximately 70 percent of your previous results. If you lost 20 pounds during the first six weeks, then you'll likely lose 14 pounds during the second six weeks. If you have 40 pounds or more to lose, you may have to commit for three, four, or more six-week sessions.

The key is to turn your week-by-week eating, superhydrating, and Bowflex training into week-by-week steps that move you closer to your goal.

REPEAT THE EATING PLAN

The eating plans for women appear in chapters 20, 22, and 23. They are similar enough that they can be interchanged. The eating plans for men are in chapter 20 and chapter 23. Chapter 21 applies to athletes and other individuals who require higher energy levels—so do not interchange that eating plan with the others.

Personally, I'm partial to the descending-calorie approach in chapter 20, The Body-Leanness Plan. I've seen it repeated by many individuals for as long as six months. Whether you descend your calories or keep them at a constant level, be sure you have a plan and, most important, adhere to it with discipline.

The eating plan does get easier the second time around because you're more familiar with the menus and foods. You'll be much better now at judging serving sizes without having to weigh and measure everything. You'll also be more efficient in your shopping, cooking, and preparation time.

Sooner or later, however, you're going to have to deal with holidays and all the high-calorie foods that traditionally surround them.

COMBAT HOLIDAY EATING

Birthdays, Thanksgiving, Christmas, New Year's, Valentine's Day, Easter, Mother's Day, Father's Day, July Fourth, and Labor Day all involve festive eating and drinking—usually in excess. Here are seven steps to help you take charge during these situations:

Plan ahead, eat ahead. Find out what is on the menu. If there are not enough low-calorie choices, eat at home—not an entire meal but a healthy 200- to 300-calorie snack. That way you won't be so tempted and overwhelmed when the meal begins.

Limit alcohol consumption. Alcohol is calorie dense. It also tends to cloud your ability to forgo other high-calorie foods. Stick to sparkling water or plain water and ice.

Try to eat something sweet initially. No you don't have to eat your dessert first, although doing so would probably help. Something sweet—fruit is great, especially pineapple, or perhaps two bite-size samples of Aunt Sally's fruit cobbler—will elevate your blood sugar level in about 20 minutes. With the correct timing, when the main part of the meal is served, your appetite will already be partially curbed.

Load up on green salads. Green salads are low in calories as long as the dressing is handled with care. If possible, get yours without dressing and add something light and low in calories.

Go easy on the meat and avoid the gravy. "Two slices, please" should be your motto. White turkey breast is best, with no gravy.

Say no gracefully. You can flatter Aunt Sally by telling her how delicious a particular high-calorie food looks—then ask for the recipe.

Skip dessert, almost. If you can't skip dessert, ask for a small serving and limit it to two bites.

In spite of the above steps, if you still consumed more than you should (let's face it, we're all human), then there are still a couple of things you can do.

First, get up from the table and get active. Perhaps you can take a walk around the block and encourage others to join you. Maybe you can shoot baskets out

DINING OUT WHILE DIETING

Dining out doesn't have to be damaging to your diet. If you have to eat at a restaurant while you're trying to lose or maintain weight, here are the best rules to follow:

- Request that a large pitcher of ice water be placed on your table. Drink freely before, during, and after the meal.
- Don't open the menu. The menu is supposed to entice you to spend big, and most restaurants know how to sell their rich, expensive specialties.
- Choose a simple green salad without such garnishes as croutons and bacon bits. Lemon juice, vinegar, or low-fat dressing is preferable to any creamy or oily dressing.
- Select one or two vegetables with nothing added. A plain baked potato is nearly always available. Other good choices are broccoli, cauliflower, and carrots.

- Ask the waiter what kind of fresh fish is in the kitchen. Though chicken breast is acceptable, you're better off with fish, which is always cooked to order. Because of its lengthier preparation time, chicken is usually prepared earlier in the day with various marinades and sauces.
- Order a whitefish and have it baked, steamed, or broiled with nothing on it.
- Be very specific with your order. Double-check to make certain that your waiter understands exactly what you want. Don't be afraid to send something back if it's not what you requested.
- Have decaffeinated coffee or tea for dessert, or at most some fresh strawberries or raspberries.
- Reinforce the waiter and the manager as you leave. Make them aware of your special likes and dislikes about the food and the service.

back with some of the kids. Or, if nothing else, you can volunteer to help clean up the kitchen, which could require some significant calories.

Second, if you do overeat, don't swear off food for the rest of the day. Doing so simply forces your body to think something is wrong, and it resorts to fat storage as a means of survival. Instead, feed your body a small meal three hours later and again in another three hours. The following day, get back on your planned menus.

CONTINUE YOUR BOWFLEX TRAINING

If you commit to another six-week program, you may be tempted to perform more than the recommended ten Bowflex exercises that you did during Weeks 5 and 6 the first time around. Or maybe you'd like to do more sets on each exercise than the recommended one set. It's okay to be tempted, but don't give in. More exercises than ten and more sets than one are not a better system of training. Too much exercise, especially if you are on a reduced-calorie diet, places too much stress on your recovery ability. As a result, you will curb your muscle growth and stunt your fat loss.

Stay with ten Bowflex exercises for your second six

weeks. You can, however, make a few exercise substitutions—just enough to add a little variety. If you're interested in doing this, review chapters 6, 7, and 8, and make the appropriate modifications. Be sure and keep written records of your substitutions. But you don't have to modify any of the routines. You can certainly keep performing the same exercises and routines for the second six weeks—and many people prefer doing just that.

Your job on each Bowflex exercise stays the same: *do 8 to 12 repetitions, always attempting one more, with as much resistance on the Power Rods as possible while maintaining good form.* Again, how you do each exercise is much more important than the amount and variety of the exercises.

EXTEND OTHER PRACTICES

Along with your reduced-calorie eating and Bowflex training, your other practices—such as superhydration, moderate walking, thermodynamics, and extra resting—should remain at the same level for the second six weeks as they were at the end of your first six-week program.

Achieving your goals is only weeks away. Stay on course.

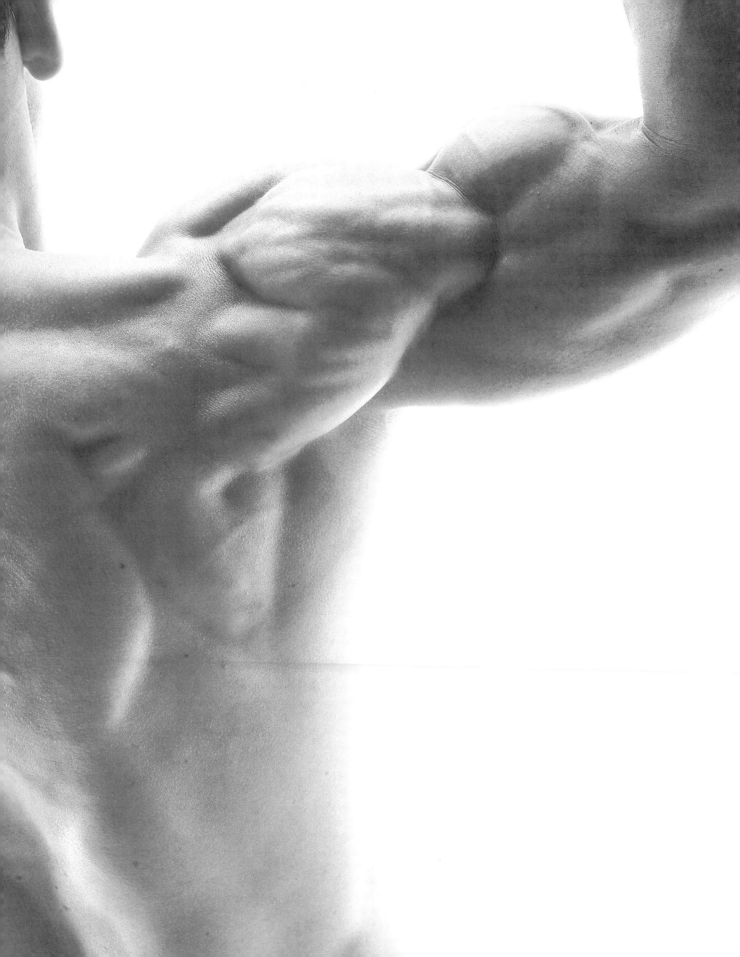

28

MAINTENANCE:

MODIFYING KEY FACTORS

MOST PEOPLE WHO DILIGENTLY APPLY the Bowflex fat-loss plans eventually reach their goals. Then, the objective becomes maintenance. Successful maintenance eases you into eating slightly more calories and larger portions week by week.

But beware. One of the historical problems with maintaining weight loss is that once the strict calorie counting is relaxed, most people underestimate the calories they consume. For example, researchers at St. Luke's–Roosevelt Hospital Center and Columbia University in New York City had dieters keep journals of how much they ate. Then, they compared those records with sophisticated laboratory tests that accurately measured each morsel of food they consumed. The result: The dieters underreported their food intake by an average of 47 percent.

Their exercise journals were even worse. Analyzing the dieters' physical-activity claims versus what they actually did was overreported by 51 percent.

In other words, most people who successfully lose their targeted amount of fat, left to their own eyeballing techniques, will underestimate the number of calories they eat each day and overestimate their exercise levels.

Based on my own experience, I tend to agree with these findings, although perhaps not to the same degree. But I have seen that most dieters tend to misjudge their eating and exercising. I've observed many of my successful participants, during their maintenance phase, add back too many calories too quickly while reducing the intensity of their strength training. The end result is that they start gaining fat and losing muscle—bit by bit, day by day, week by week until they realize that they've regained about half of what they'd lost, and lost about half of what they'd built!

Do not let such things happen to you. Understand now that most of us have the tendency to underestimate our eating and overestimate our exercising. When we do that what we're trying to do is to defy the laws of thermodynamics, or get something for nothing, which doesn't work.

Maintenance boils down to the same discipline, motivation, and patience that got you through the fat-loss and muscle-building programs initially. There are, however, a few minor adjustments that you must understand and apply.

FOLLOW A CARBOHYDRATE-RICH, MODERATE-CALORIE EATING PLAN

Carbohydrate-rich meals are a staple in fat loss, maintenance, and healthy eating. Remember that

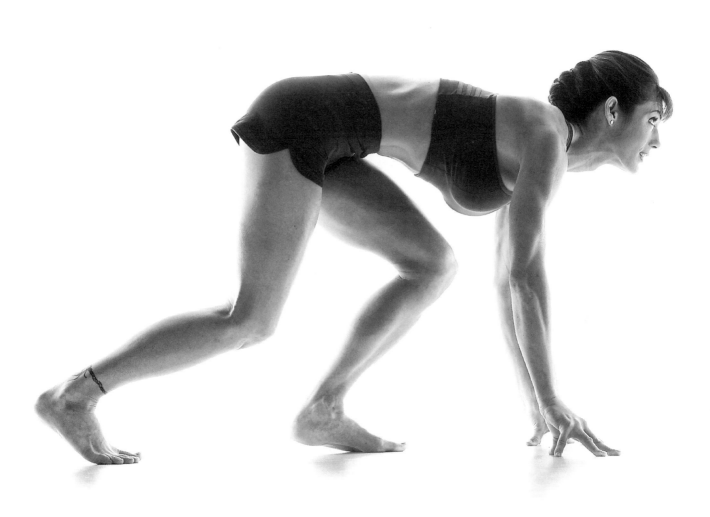

fruits, vegetables, breads, and cereals are your primary sources of carbohydrates. During maintenance, however, you'll be progressing from low calories each day to moderate calories. Generally, a middle-aged man of average height and weight should be able to maintain his weight on between 1,800 and 2,400 calories a day. An average middle-aged woman can do so on between 1,400 and 2,000 calories a day.

Athletes and other fitness-minded people who have been through the Hard-Body Challenge would need to add 300 to 400 calories to the range: 2,200 to 2,800 for men and 1,700 to 2,300 for women.

You can figure out the maintenance level best for you by gradually adding calories back into your eating plan. Remember, it's important to be accurate in your calorie counting. Read labels. Accurately weigh and measure your food and keep records of what you eat along with their calorie counts. Stay at your initial maintenance level of calories for a week. If you are still losing weight, raise the level by 100 calories a day for the next seven days. In another week or two, your body weight will stabilize. You'll know then that you've reached your upper limit of your maintenance calorie level.

Several pocket-sized manuals are available that contain nutritional information on many foods. It's a good idea to use one in your shopping.

EAT SMALLER MEALS MORE FREQUENTLY

During the programs contained in this book, you've been limiting yourself to five or six small meals a day of 500 calories or less. To maintain your body weight, set the limit at 600 calories for a man and 500 calories for a woman. Sometimes a few extra calories during a meal are acceptable, but be very careful. You should know by now that all calories count—PERIOD—and that large meals are especially problematic. Keep all your meals small and you'll be well ahead.

SUPERHYDRATE EACH DAY

By now, you should have experienced firsthand the power of superhydration and its importance in fat loss, muscle building, internal and external cooling, and skin health. Water supports your every function. Make your water bottle, and the sipping of 1 gallon of ice-cold fluid from it each day, a permanent fixture in your new lifestyle.

STRENGTH TRAIN TWICE A WEEK

Don't let your newly built muscles wither away. To prevent this, you've got to continue with your Bowflex training. Stronger muscles are an insurance policy against regaining fat. Once your muscles begin shrinking from lack of work, your lost fat will gradually start to return. I repeat: Don't let this happen.

The primary difference between muscle building and muscle maintenance is that you don't need to train as often. You may reduce your frequency from three times per week to two. For example, instead of working out on Monday, Wednesday, and Friday, go to a Monday-Thursday schedule.

Keep in mind that more Bowflex strength training is not necessarily better. Better strength training is harder. And harder means less. Apply this concept for the rest of your life and your strength and leanness may well exceed your goals.

PRACTICE A FEW OTHER ACTIONS AS NEEDED

Any of the other actions recommended throughout this book, such as moderate walking, staying cool, and getting extra rest and sleep, can be reinstated in your maintenance schedule anytime you need a boost. Believe me, from time to time, you will need a boost.

Will you ever reach a state of completion where you won't need a boost? I doubt it. If it did happen, however, it would be as a result of repeated practice.

A STORY RELATED TO REPEATED PRACTICE

A good friend of mine, who is an Orlando Magic basketball fan, claims he witnessed an interesting scenario in 1990 prior to an Orlando–Boston Celtics game. Larry Bird, the superstar for the Celtics, was warming up at one end of the court in his typical way. He has a rolling metal rack with two tiers and eight basketballs by his side and a couple of boys to retrieve the balls and keep the coaster full. Bird practices shooting from all around the basket—and he likes to shoot fast, hence the rolling ball rack and the boys to keep it full.

A small crowd of about twenty-five people soon congregates in the stands to watch him. He's in his zone—oblivious to what's going on around him—nothing except the balls and the basket. Soon, however, there's a loudmouthed heckler—a fifty-year-old man wearing a baseball hat—who keeps challenging Bird.

"Hey, Bird, let's see your hook shot!"

"How about a jumper from the top of the circle?"

"Can you still do a one-handed set shot?"

Nothing from Bird. Not even a look, nod, or response. Nothing except net, as Bird hits from all over the court. He rarely misses two times in a row. The heckler then opens his wallet and pulls out a twenty-dollar bill. "Hey, Bird," he shouts, "here's twenty bucks, if you can make three straight from the corner."

No response at all from Bird.

"Bird, you're chicken. You're afraid to bet, right?"

Still nothing.

"I guess you're over the hill. Just can't take the pressure anymore. That's it, isn't it?"

That finally got Bird's attention, which delighted the heckler. "Hey, Bird, twenty dollars says you can't make three straight from the corner." Then he paused as Bird made eye contact with him and walked toward the corner with his ball rack in tow, and then the guy hollered, "Left-handed."

Bird replied calmly, "Left-handed," knowing that since he's right-handed he'd been suckered into an awkward bet.

"Tell you what," Bird responded, "Let's make that bet a hundred dollars."

All eyes were on the heckler as he paused, swallowed hard, and agreed.

Suddenly, Bird was in the corner and, with his left hand, let fly three balls so fast that they were all in the air at the same time and with the same result: *swish, swish, swish!*

Larry Bird walked over, grabbed the guy's $100, smiled, and jogged off the court to the howls of the spectators. Even the heckler, who had just lost $100, was absolutely amazed.

Repeated practice, especially if the practice leads to better skills, is essential for success. But Larry Bird's three successful shots from the corner, left-handed, with $100 riding on the outcome, goes beyond repeated practice. Bird's success is directly related to what is called *overlearning*. Overlearning, from my more than forty years of study, is the single most relevant factor in helping people maintain their fat loss.

OVERLEARNING AND LONG-TERM SUCCESS

Overlearning means practice beyond goal achievement. Larry Bird has surely shot the ball at the basket not thousands of times but probably at least a million times. Since Bird played basketball for thirty years, a million shots amounts to ninety-one shots a day. Yes, ninety-one shots a day at a basket, every day for thirty years, would probably make anyone more proficient at shooting a basketball, and Larry Bird did that several times over!

Overlearning is a primary reason why Larry Bird was such a superior shooter. He could have probably come close to making all three of those corner shots blindfolded.

Overlearning, as it relates to *The Bowflex Body Plan*, means practicing certain behaviors again and again until they are so ingrained that almost nothing can disturb them. Overlearning produces automatic actions. Without thinking, you respond with the correct behavior. The more times you experience the desired response, the better you get and the more lasting the pattern becomes.

As I look back closely at the thousands of people who've been through my fat-loss programs, the ones who have kept their fat off have done so because of overlearning. The practices, such as eating smaller meals more frequently, superhydrating your system, and keeping your muscles strong, have become fundamental lifestyle changes. They are repeated daily and weekly, just like brushing your teeth without a second thought.

How long does it take to overlearn?

EIGHTY-FOUR DAYS TO OVERLEARNING

The good news is that overlearning doesn't take thirty years. In fact, it requires a lot less. The bad news is that overlearning, as you might expect, is still very challenging.

I've observed with my participants that it takes approximately twenty-one days to establish a pattern and eighty-four days to make that pattern automatic. In other words, my fat-loss plans get easier for most after three weeks. If they continue with the plan for twelve weeks, or eighty-four days, their daily actions become almost automatic.

Twelve weeks? No problem, you might be thinking.

Here's the kicker: Psychologists who study overlearning believe that an eighty-four-day time span of behavior modification means eighty-four *consecutive* days. If you practice the discipline for twenty-eight days, forty-two days, seventy days, or even eighty-two days and break the pattern on the next day, then you must start over.

That's why it is so hard for many people to keep the fat off permanently. That's also why those fat-loss programs that allow you to break your diet and cheat one day a week don't work well in the long term. Cheating for "just one day" simply means it will be much easier for you to cheat on another day. Soon the cheat days will outnumber the diet days.

I've observed, once again, that participants who go through one of my six-week programs twice (which amounts to eighty-four consecutive days), if they do so without cheating a single day, have the greatest probability of long-term success.

In spite of financial problems, difficulties with their children, divorce, and serious accidents, the vast majority of these people do not regain their lost fat. It's not because their lost weight is more important than such tragedies—far from it—but the habits ac-quired through overlearning are so deeply ingrained that they persist even when stressful events come to the forefront.

Take charge of your life now—with overlearning.

THE POWER LIVES!

With *The Bowflex Body Plan*, you can lose fat and build muscle efficiently and effectively. With an understanding and application of the guidelines in this chapter, you can now keep your lost fat off and newly built muscles intact.

Twelve weeks, or eighty-four days, shouldn't be too much to ask of anyone. Just check with Larry Bird or any of the Bowflex superstars you see in the television advertisements.

Keep the power in your corner. Keep the power alive.

29
QUESTIONS, PLEASE:

UP-TO-DATE ANSWERS
TO PREVALENT PROBLEMS

AS YOU CAN PROBABLY IMAGINE, most of the questions I receive relate to my fat-loss programs. Here's a roundup of the most common concerns and my answers.

FRESH VERSUS FROZEN BAGELS

Q: For breakfast on the Body-Leanness Plan, can I substitute a fresh bagel from my local deli for the recommended frozen variety?

A: Though a fresh bagel is tasty, the problem is that most deli bagels contain well over the 210 calories of a frozen bagel. A 1996 report that analyzed bagels from more than a dozen New York City bakers found that not one supplied less than 250 calories. Interestingly, some of the bagels were advertised as being low in calories while they actually supplied from 500 to 600 calories each. Stick to the frozen bagels for breakfast. You can be sure of their calorie count.

SWITCHING LUNCH AND DINNER

Q: May I have my dinner for lunch and my lunch for dinner?

A: Yes.

MORE CALORIES FOR A LARGE MAN

Q: I'm a twenty-seven-year-old man. I weigh 300 pounds at a height of 6 feet 5 inches. Because of my well-above-average weight and height, do I need to do anything different on the eating part of the Body-Leanness Plan?

A: Most men who are over 6 feet 2 inches tall and weigh more than 250 pounds—or men who are extremely active or work outdoors in jobs such as construction, loading and unloading, or plumbing—require an extra 300 calories per day. Usually, I recommend that such people add 300 calories worth of whole-wheat bread, spread throughout their meals, to the total. Since you're taller and heavier than that, I recommend that you adhere to the Hard-Body Eating Plan in chapter 21. It supplies approximately 1,900 calories a day, which should work well for you.

FAVORITE FAMILY RECIPES

Q: The frozen microwave meals have been a real help for me and my husband. But after six weeks, he wants me to go back to some of our favorite recipes from our pre-dieting days. I'm afraid because I know many of them are loaded with calories. What should I do?

A: Food-science research reveals that the typical American family tends to eat from the same ten recipes repeatedly. Your mission, then, is to adapt those recipes with an eye toward leanness. Here are some hints:

• Challenge every ingredient one by one. Fat-free milk, not whole. Two egg whites instead of an entire egg. Ground turkey in place of ground beef. Seasonings, such as onion, garlic, and herbs, as well as some tomato and green pepper, will spice up ground turkey so you won't miss ground beef.

• Replace sour cream in dips and toppings with a cup of low-fat cottage cheese whirled in a blender with one tablespoon of fresh lemon juice. Plain low-fat yogurt or buttermilk can be substituted for sour cream in salad dressings and baked goods.

• Buy reduced-calorie light mayonnaise, or make your own with half mayonnaise and half low-fat yogurt.

• Make soups and stews a day in advance so you can chill them and remove fat from the top before reheating and serving.

• Cut gravy calories by using arrowroot, cornstarch, or flour to thicken pan drippings rather than a butter-drenched roux.

• Use nonstick skillets, or vegetable oil cooking spray, instead of traditional pan frying.

This sprinkling of suggestions and substitutions is only a start. Developing ten lean recipes based on your established family favorites is well worth the effort.

HEADACHES FROM 1,000 CALORIES

Q: I often get headaches when I eat only 1,000 calories a day. What should I do?

A: Your headaches may be caused by going longer than three hours between meals or snacks. Try spacing your eating episodes closer together.

Also, some people who are used to drinking regular coffee with caffeine get headaches when they stop drinking coffee for several days. If this is the case, ease off the coffee more gradually.

HEADACHES FROM COLD WATER

Q: Sometimes I get a headache when I drink ice-cold water. Can I drink the water without it being chilled?

A: Yes, but you won't get the 123-calories-per-gallon thermogenic effect from warming the cold water to core body temperature. Try a more gradual drinking (sipping with a large straw is best) of the water. You may have been consuming it too quickly.

BRUISES ON THIGHS

Q: I'm a middle-aged woman who gets black and blue marks on my legs when I diet. Am I doing something wrong?

A: I doubt you are doing anything wrong. Such black and blue marks are usually the result of increased estrogen circulating in your body, which weakens the walls of the capillaries and causes them to break under the slightest pressure. When this happens, blood escapes and a bruise occurs. Estrogen is broken down in the liver, and so is fat. When you are dieting, your liver breaks down the fat, leaving a lot more estrogen in the bloodstream.

It may be helpful to supplement your diet with a little extra vitamin C, 100 milligrams per day, to help toughen the walls of the capillaries.

TEENAGE SON AND DAUGHTER NEED TO LOSE FAT

Q: I'm a forty-year-old woman with a teenage son and daughter. My husband and I both want to lose 10 pounds and the children would also like to lose some weight. Can the whole family go through the Body-Leanness Plan?

A: It would be great if the whole family could do the eating plan together, but you cannot. The number of calories per day is the problem. Teenagers require significantly more calories each day than 1,500, which is the highest level in the eating plans. Check with a registered dietician (RD) for appropriate recommendations for your children.

Your teenage son and daughter could, however, certainly follow the Bowflex training routines. Make certain they are supervised and that they practice the exercises seriously.

BACKSLIDING FORWARD

Q: I messed up on the recommended eating plan last week and I think I put back a few pounds. What should I do?

A: There's no disgrace in backsliding. The disgrace lies in letting a lapse get you so discouraged that you quit trying. Don't let yourself fall into this destructive trap. True control and true power revolve around the realization that permanent fat loss is a long-term project that is bound to have ups and downs. You're feeling down now. Get back on your eating plan and move forward.

STRENGTH TRAINING ON THE ROAD

Q: When I travel, which I do frequently, I want to continue with my strength training. Should I use the hotel's exercise equipment or should I plan to visit a fitness center? More importantly, what exercises should I do?

A: It's great that you want to strength train while on the road. Many hotels have exercise rooms that usually contain a multistation gym of some sort. If that's the case, then there's no reason to visit a fitness center. You should be able to generalize from your familiar Bowflex exercises to those provided by a multistation machine. Make sure you first read the exercise instructions attached to the machine or displayed on a nearby wall chart. I recommend that you perform the Leg Curl, Leg Extension, Leg Press, Calf Raise, Bench Press, Lat Pulldown, Seated Press, and Biceps Curl. Then, you can finish off with some form of an abdominal exercise, such as the trunk curl or reverse trunk curl.

If your hotel has no exercise room, then ask the manager at the front desk for the phone number of a nearby fitness center. Many hotels and motels will have already established a relationship with a local club. Make the call and ask what the requirements are for gaining a guest pass. If you decide to visit the club, then I'd recommend doing something similar to the previously listed routine: one set of 8 to 12 repetitions of four lower-body exercises combined with four upper-body exercises.

Visiting a strange fitness center is not the time to experiment. Keep your workout simple. Get in, work out, and leave.

WORKING THE LOWER ABS

Q: When I do the Bowflex Abdominal Crunch, I feel it in my upper abs. I need to work my lower abs, too. What can I do for them?

A: If you're doing the Seated Abdominal Crunch correctly, you are working your lower abdominal muscles, but you will never feel the effect in your lower abdominal muscles as you do in the upper area. Here's why:

First, the largest section of your abdominal muscles is high on your waist, under your rib cage, not

BARRY OZER'S RESULTS

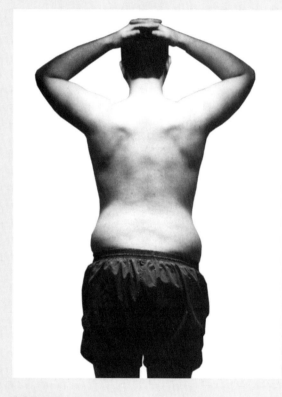
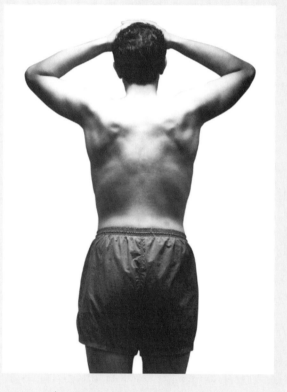

AGE: **25**
HEIGHT: **6'2"**
BEFORE WEIGHT: **239¼ POUNDS**
BEFORE WAIST SIZE: **44⅜"**

- Lost **71¼ pounds** of fat in eighteen weeks
- Built **5½ pounds** of muscle
- Trimmed **13¾"** off waist

low or beneath your navel. You always feel abdominal exercises most in the mass of the muscles and toward the origin.

Second, the long, paired rectus abdominis muscles originate under your rib cage and insert into your pelvis. But when these muscles get near the region of your navel, they actually plunge through an opening in the horizontally crossing transversus abdominis muscles. The transversus abdominis, which lies on top of the insertion point of the rectus abdominis, tends to reduce the sensitivity of the deeper rectus abdominis.

Third, muscles begin to contract at the ends, where the tendons attach to the bones, and move gradually toward the center. Thus, to work the portion of the rectus abdominis that inserts on the pelvis, you have to move very slowly at the beginning of each repetition of the Seated Abdominal Crunch. Since the abdominal crunch is a short-range movement, it's easy to cheat at the beginning. Don't let this happen. Focus intensely on the start and you'll feel the exercise more in your lower area, especially as you get stronger and apply more resistance.

Fourth, sometimes bringing the iliopsoas muscles—which connect to your spine and thigh bones and lie underneath the abdominal muscles—into action can synergize feeling in the region below the navel. If you are strong enough, in your lower back as well as your abdominals, you may want to try hooking your feet under the legs of the Bowflex machine, which will allow you to increase the range of movement of the abdominal crunch by several inches. Move carefully as you try this version.

Fifth, many people confuse working their lower abdominals with the removal of fatty deposits below the navel. Remember, working the lower abdominals does not draw calories from fat that may lie near the involved muscles. Spot reduction of fat is not possible.

HELP FOR LOVE HANDLES

Q: I'm a forty-two-year-old man. My body fat seems to be thickest over my sides. Can I ever get rid of these so-called love handles, which I certainly don't love?

A: I understand what you're talking about. Many men store fat first on the sides of their waist, which means it will be the last to come off. *First on, last off* is one of the basic principles of fat deposition and reduction.

I want you to look at the before and after photos of Barry Ozer on the opposite page. He was in my first Bowflex study in 1995 at Gainesville. The time between the photos was eighteen weeks. Ozer had some of the thickest love handles that I've ever seen. But they didn't start shrinking significantly until the thirteenth week. By the end of the eighteenth week—and after a reduction of 13¾ inches from his waist—his love handles had shrunk to the point that they were unnoticeable.

So, yes, you can get rid of your love handles. Even if it takes you eighteen weeks, you can do it.

NO LEG EXTENSION

Q: I don't have the Leg-Extension/Leg-Curl Attachment with my Bowflex machine. I know I can substitute the

Seated Leg Curl for the Prone Leg Curl, but what can I substitute for the Leg Extension?

A: Instead of the Leg Extension, use the Wall Squat that I describe on page 213.

PREGNANCY AND BOWFLEX TRAINING

Q: I've been exercising on Bowflex for almost a year now and I really like it. Just two days ago, I found out that I'm two months pregnant. Can I continue to use my same Bowflex routines? Should I be doing anything differently?

A: You'll probably be able to continue your Bowflex routines, with certain modifications, which I'll discuss. But first, there's some exciting new research related to pregnancy and strength training that I'd like to share with you.

Throughout pregnancy the body produces hormones that relax and contract the muscles of the uterus, abdomen, buttocks, thighs, and lower back during the birth. If these muscles are strong and in good condition, a woman will have an easier time at birth. Also, she will feel and look better before and after the baby is born.

Prior to birth, especially during the last trimester, there is extra stress and strain on certain muscles. Many women tilt their pelvic area forward and bend the upper part of their bodies backward to compensate for the weight of the heavy uterus. As a result, backaches frequently develop. As breasts become larger, additional stress is placed on the chest, the shoulders, and the upper back. The Bowflex upper-body exercises are particularly good for a pregnant woman because they minimize uneven forces on the joints and maximize muscular strength.

There is also a slowing of the bloodflow in the lower extremities during pregnancy. Many times this can cause stagnation of the blood in the legs, leading to varicose veins. The Bowflex lower-body exercises can definitely improve circulation.

The needs of pregnancy put an added burden on a mother's heart. Not only can Bowflex exercise increase the heart's efficiency, but research shows that exercise by a woman during pregnancy will increase the strength of the unborn baby's heart.

Take this book with you for your next doctor's appointment. Show your doctor exactly what you've been doing. With his or her approval—which is very important—you'll probably be able to continue at your same level of intensity as long as your pregnancy runs a normal and healthy course.

Midway through your pregnancy, there are certain exercise positions on a Bowflex machine that could cause complications. Anytime you have to lie flat on your back for several minutes could cause undue stress on the fetus. The Lying Shoulder Pullover, Lying Lat Pulldown, Lying Biceps Curl, and Lying Triceps Extension are examples. I would not do these exercises. Also, the enlarging uterus will preclude you from doing the Prone Leg Curl. Instead, do the Seated Leg Curl. Most of the other Bowflex exercises can be used regularly throughout pregnancy.

According to Dr. Mona Shangold, a well-known sports gynecologist, the following warning signs are cause for immediate evaluation and the cessation of training: pain, bleeding, rupture of membranes, and absence of fetal movement. If you experience any of these complications, call your physician right away. Do not resume your exercise until you have your doctor's approval.

BODYBUILDING WITH BOWFLEX

Q: I'm heavily into bodybuilding and I can't believe that Bowflex can build a thick chest and big arms, like you promise with your blitzes. Shoot straight with me: Don't you really have to lift free weights to get a really thick chest and really big arms?

A: If you have the genetic potential to build a really thick chest and really big arms, then you can certainly get them with Bowflex. Bowflex may not have the macho image that goes with doing a 300-pound bench press with a barbell, but I guarantee you that 300 pounds of Power Rods on a Bowflex machine will stimulate your chest to grow in a similar manner.

I, too, was heavily into bodybuilding for many years. When Nautilus machines came onto the scene in 1970, most bodybuilders believed that Nautilus was inferior to free weights. Rather than accept a tool that could help them get bigger and stronger, they rejected it because it was different from what they were used to doing. If, on the other hand, you persuaded the bodybuilders to try Nautilus for just a few exercises, then many of them responded positively.

Now, more than thirty years later, most bodybuilders use a combination of free weights and machines. There are certain body parts that are impossible to isolate without heavy-duty machines. But Bowflex is not classified as a heavy-duty machine and it doesn't contain a 300-pound weight stack. So it's no wonder that most bodybuilders today reject Bowflex. It's different from what they are used to doing.

If that's the case with you, then I challenge you to try Bowflex. In fact, apply the arm exercises that make up the Bigger-Arms Blitz. I'm predicting that you're going to be very surprised at how the machine operates—as well as how your triceps and biceps will feel during and after the exercises.

ADDING CREATINE

Q: Since creatine helps with the muscle-building process, is it okay if I add it to the Body-Leanness Plan? Wouldn't this help the entire process of losing fat and building muscle simultaneously?

A: In fact, I tried doing exactly that with myself, as well as with three athletes. The results were poor.

Creatine seems to deter fat loss. It makes it much harder for the reduced-calorie diet to do its job. On the other hand, if you're trying to build as much muscle as possible, creatine helps, along with a higher-calorie diet.

So use creatine with the Thicker-Chest Blitz and the Bigger-Arms Blitz, or in a strictly muscle-building program, but don't apply it with the Body-Leanness Plan or the other fat-loss courses in this book.

KEEPING THE FAT OFF

Q: I lost 46½ pounds on The Body-Leanness Plan and I've kept it off for almost six months. Can I ever go back to eating the way I once did?

A: If "eating the way you once did" means consuming 1,000 or more calories for most meals, mixed with high-calorie snacks and rich desserts, then probably not. Do you truly want to return to eating the way you once did?

You should be able to gradually add some calories back to your meals. Maybe you've already done this, your body weight has stabilized, and you're telling me that you still want more food—or at the very least you still *think about* wanting more food.

Some experts who deal exclusively with obesity believe that you've got to keep that lost weight off for a minimum of one year to reestablish your body's chemistry or set point. Other experts bump that time period from one year to two years. Yet others extend the time to more than three years. They all agree, however, that the longer you keep it off, the higher the probability of keeping it off per-

294 Pounds of Fat Lost in Six Weeks

Five women and nine men, ages twenty-five to fifty-six, from the Portland, Oregon, area volunteered to participate in the Bowflex Challenge. The project was supervised by Glen Baggerly, owner of The Gym in Portland.

Both the women and the men applied the Body-Leanness Plan, as described in chapter 20, for the duration of the study, from June 12 to July 24, 2002.

In six weeks, these fourteen people lost 294 pounds of fat, or about 21 pounds per person. In addition, each participant trimmed an average of 5⅜ inches from his or her waist.

Why not do for yourself what individuals such as Sha, Alex, James, and Becky did for their bodies—in just six weeks? Accept the Bowflex Challenge—*now*.

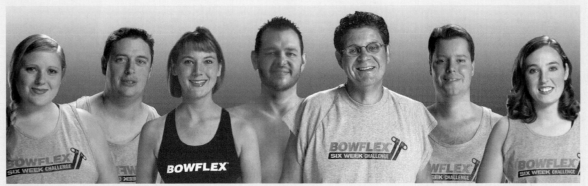

Sha Boland	Art Gailey	Sherrie Wilhelmi	Alex Bejarano	Larry Marceaux	Kory Hutchinson	Melia Fisher
−23.75 lbs	−22 lbs	−6 lbs	−34.5 lbs	−28 lbs	−32 lbs	−9.5 lbs

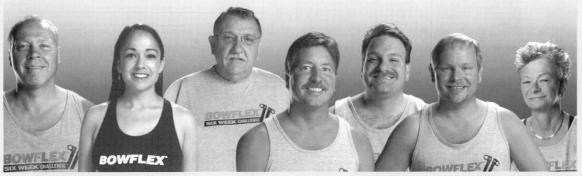

James Hoover	Michelle Sandoval	Terry Stewart	Brian Lewis	Steve Ruscigno	Brian Strandberg	Becky Goodford
−34.5 lbs	−6.25 lbs	−33 lbs	−15 lbs	−19.5 lbs	−16.25 lbs	−13.75 lbs

manently, which relates to the concept of over-learning.

I believe that much of the eating-more answer lies in elevating your basal metabolic rate. The best way to do this is to add as much muscle as you can to your body. Don't be satisfied with 3 or 4 pounds in six weeks. Keep working. Try to build another 3 or 4 pounds, and then another 3 or 4 pounds.

I think the average untrained man can add from 12 to 16 pounds of muscle to his body before he reaches his genetic potential. The typical untrained woman can add from 6 to 9 pounds to her body. Don't forget, a pound of muscle forces your metabolism to rise 37.5 calories. Said another way, 10 pounds of new muscle means you can consume an extra 375 calories each day.

So, my advice is as follows:

• Continue to eat moderate-sized meals, that is, fewer than 600 calories.

• Work diligently at keeping your lost fat off for at least a year.

• Understand that keeping it off for two years is better than one year and three years is better than two years.

• Build more and more muscle.

SENSITIVITY TO COLD

Q: After losing 12 pounds, I seem to be extra sensitive to feeling cold most of the time. Why?

A: Some women and men who progress through the fat-loss programs often complain of being cold. Even during the summer, air-conditioning can bring on the chills. So can the ice-cold water used in superhydration.

Much of the fat on your body is located right under the skin and acts as insulation. Once you thin this insulation, it's no wonder that you become more sensitive to cold. Your fingers, toes, and even the tip of your nose can be affected.

If you still have more fat to lose, then you're in the mode to do so very efficiently. Rather than put on a coat or sweater, remember that the state of almost shivering is one of the best ways to burn calories. Move around, take a walk, and try to keep that sweater off a little longer. You can train your body to generate its own heat by burning more body fat.

The other thing that you can do to generate more heat is to add another pound or two of muscle. Perhaps you've already added 3 to 4 pounds. Don't be satisfied. Up the intensity of your workouts and experiment with some advanced techniques.

IN CONTROL AND LIKING IT!

Q: I'm amazed at how much better my business associates treat me now that I've lost most of my excessive fat. What's happening here?

A: You're absolutely right. Many of the successful participants that I've worked with have made similar comments. Rightfully or wrongfully, a lean physique tells the world that discipline and motivation reside within. True or not, it matters little because the perception might as well be reality.

First impressions are certainly not everything, but a poor one sure takes a long time to overcome. No matter how smart, sincere, or responsible you are, your appearance acts as a filter through which almost everything else is judged.

Physiology speaks even before you do. If anything the least bit articulate comes out of the mouth of a lean body, the intelligence is assessed in glowing terms.

Sadly, the same words spoken by someone who is overfat don't land with as much impact. The person doing the encountering would be skeptical, thinking perhaps, "If this person's so sharp, why doesn't he or she do something to lose weight?"

Your appearance can be an asset or a liability, or maybe it's just neutral. You don't have to become obsessed with winning a contest based on looks. The right business suit is a great equalizer, so long as the body inside is within shooting distance of its ideal body-fat level.

Getting a leaner, stronger body puts you in control of your own destiny. You should expect more good things to happen to you in the future.

30
A PRESCRIPTION FOR LIFE:

THE POWER IS YOURS—
TODAY, TOMORROW, & FOREVER!

"IF I'D HAVE KNOWN I WAS GOING to live this long, I would've taken better care of myself."

That adage sounds like something Dean Martin, Jackie Gleason, or Groucho Marx might have said, but it was actually from jazz pianist Eubie Blake. Unlike a lot of comedians, who are entertaining but lead melancholic lives, Blake must have done quite a few things right because he lived to be one hundred. Still, in retrospect, I'll bet Eubie—as well as Dean, Jackie, and Groucho—wished he had taken better care of himself.

Nothing is more destructive to the health of a person than a loss of passion. Unfortunately, as many people age their enthusiasm evaporates and they gradually withdraw from society. Or, as Helen Keller once put it, "Science may have found a cure for most evils; but it has no remedy for the worst of them all—the apathy of human beings."

Each man and woman reading this chapter should, right now, STOP.

Reflect for a few moments and realize that your life and most everything connected to it slip away much faster than you ever anticipate. Don't take your health for granted or assume that your pains and ailments are normal. Reevaluate, if necessary, and renew your motivation.

If you haven't already decided to take better care of your body, decide now and start today. There's a Bowflex plan in this book that provides the right prescription for your body.

COMBATING THE PHYSIOLOGICAL FACTORS OF AGING

Muscular strength, the most important component of physical fitness, is also the most important component in combating the aging process.

According to Drs. William Evans and Irwin Rosenberg in their book *Biomarkers*, there are ten physiological factors associated with aging. They are as follows:

- Muscle mass

- Strength

- Basal metabolic rate

- Body-fat percentage

- Aerobic capacity

- Blood-sugar tolerance

- Cholesterol/HDL ratio

- Blood pressure

- Bone density

- The body's ability to regulate its internal temperature

Not surprising to me is that each of these factors is improved through proper strength training, the type of exercise recommended in *The Bowflex Body Plan*.

As we age, we all feel the need to take charge of our personal fitness and to understand the *why* and the *how* of what we are doing. This book supplies the information so that you can master your personal training. Furthermore, as we age there is no greater need than to keep our independence. We do not want to be dependent on others for daily care. Consistent Bowflex training is your ticket to maintaining mobility and vigorous activity and remaining independent.

STRONG MUSCLES: THE KEY

The strength of your 434 skeletal muscles produces movement from birth, makes walking possible at age one, allows running and jumping soon thereafter, and provides the basis for thousands of simple and complex actions throughout childhood and adulthood.

Somewhere between the ages of twenty to fifty, most people, through disuse and atrophy, notice a gradual decline in muscle mass and strength. This critical time span, according to Dr. Walter Bortz, marks the beginning of a long physiological death described in his book, *We Live Too Short and Die Too Long.*

With the knowledge we have today, though, we actually have a chance to do the opposite—live long and die short. With the proper Bowflex prescription, muscular weakness and flaccid shape can improve week by week, month by month, until a strong, lean body emerges.

Unto that end, the newest Bowflex machine, the Xtreme, will be available in 2004. It comes with an adjustable seat, quick-change leg extension/leg curl and lat-pulldown attachments, and a more compact footprint. It's the most integrated of the Bowflex machines, making it ideal for smaller spaces. For more details, visit www.Bowflex.com

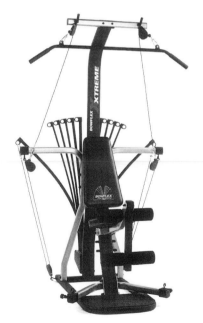

The Bowflex Xtreme, available in 2004, provides variable cable positions and multiple seat adjustments for more customized workouts.

GUIDELINES FOR LIVING LEANER AND STRONGER LONGER

Here is a brief summary of the most important principles mentioned throughout this book that you must apply to live leaner and stronger longer:

• A Bowflex machine, through bending and extending Power Rods, supplies meaningful resistance to the major muscles of your body.

• Proper strength training on a Bowflex machine involves the selection of no more than twelve exercises performed for one set of 8 to 12 repetitions and repeated progressively three times per week.

• The key to long-term success in strength training is to exercise *harder* and *briefer*.

• Consistency, not novelty, is a prelude to significant results in both strength training and nutrition.

• Eating smaller meals more often, with none of the meals exceeding 500 calories, is an important aspect of efficient fat loss.

• Superhydration, sipping at least 1 gallon of ice-cold water each day, synergizes the fat-loss and muscle-building processes.

• Extra rest and sleep, avoiding excessive stress, staying cool, and walking after your largest meal all facilitate fat loss.

• *No* is one of the strongest words in your vocabulary, especially as it relates to a reduced-calorie diet and high-calorie foods. Be proactive and use it often.

• It requires eighty-four consecutive days of practicing appropriate behaviors in eating and exercising to make the actions automatic.

• The more you overlearn the appropriate behaviors, the higher the probability that your changes will become permanent.

TRANSFORMING APPLICATIONS

By now *The Bowflex Body Plan* has made you aware of and furnished solutions for your need to:

• Build more muscle and lose more fat

• Create goals and challenges that require your action and enthusiasm

• Maintain mastery and independence as you get older

Finishing *The Bowflex Body Plan* should not be an ending for you but a beginning. The basic principles

REAL PEOPLE, REAL RESULTS

Losing Weight and Beating Diabetes

Losing significant amounts of fat can be instrumental to health, even to the point of saving a life. James D. Alexander had such an experience. Of all the people I interviewed for this book, he shed the most pounds and inches. Coincidentally, he's also the oldest at sixty-eight years of age. Alexander is a tool-and-die maker in Easley, South Carolina, and he has four grown children.

James was diagnosed as having type 2 diabetes, which can cause premature death. He also suffered from chronic lower-back pain. His doctor put him on medication and recommended that he lose significant body weight. At that time, James weighed 273 pounds at 5 feet 10 inches tall. His physician supplied him with various handouts on the correct foods to eat, which he and his wife took to heart.

"My doctor simply told me to get more exercise," James said. "Nothing specific, just more exercise. The Bowflex machine was my idea. I started using it for thirty minutes each session. And along with the diet guidelines from the doctor, I began drinking at least a gallon of ice-cold water each day."

James initiated the routine in June 2001. By Christmas, he was a different man. He was 90 pounds lighter, as his body had gone from 273 to 183 pounds.

Not lugging around all that excess fat automatically cured his nagging lower-back pain. Losing 11 inches of flab off his waist also helped. At the same time, James figured he must have gained "a bunch of muscle—maybe 5 or 6 pounds."

"As far as feeling more energetic," James replied, "before I started the program, I would have to stop and rest while walking from the parking lot to my job. Now, I run to my job—and outwork any of the younger guys there.

"I'm pleased that my new look has inspired many people I know to lose weight and to work out. Many talk to me all the time about it."

And what about the diabetes? Good news. His doctor is "very pleased." James's complications are under control and the medications are no longer necessary.

"That Bowflex machine? Yes, sir," James concluded. "I plan to use it for the rest of my life—and I figure that's going to be a long, long time."

should continue to direct you on a realistic road toward a healthier and more productive life.

I've promised you no miracles and provided no easy ways to reshape your body—*because there are none.* There are only facts—facts that translate into guidelines. Moreover, these guidelines are sometimes complicated, seldom glamorous, and often demanding. But practicing the guidelines and routines, as you have done, are the most important steps you'll ever take in your quest toward a lean, strong body.

NAUTILUS AND BOWFLEX: A GREAT TEAM

When the Nautilus headquarters was located in Lake Helen, Florida, monthly strength-training seminars for several hundred people were held for many years. The highlight of each two-day seminar was a presentation by Arthur Jones delivered at the end. Jones, with his distinctive voice, usually ranted and raved about some aspect of training, which he always made relevant to the events of the day.

"Why do we get so soon old, and so late smart?" was the way Jones began one presentation. Then, rather than employing his usual lecture voice, he quietly and passionately talked about his father, a small-town physician in Arkansas and Oklahoma, who worked long hours during the 1920s and 1930s to support his family as well as numerous relatives. Jones relived what it was like to grow up in the Oklahoma oil town of Seminole, where roughnecks, gunfighters, gamblers, and thieves seemed to be on every corner. His father treated them all, from his home office, with little payment for his efforts.

"In every sense of the word, my father was by far the best man I ever met," Jones continued, "but did I understand or appreciate his efforts at the time? Of course not. But I do now, much too late to express my appreciation." Whatever strength training is, Jones implied, it's not a replacement for family and friends.

I can't remember the rest of Jones's talk that day. But I can tell you this . . . there were a lot of dads and moms that night who received unexpected phone calls from their sons and daughters, telling them how much they were loved!

We can all learn from Jones.

Take time to acknowledge, in some special way, those who have made an impact on your life. Your parents, grandparents, siblings, maybe a teacher or two, a coach from high school, neighbors and friends—any or all may be candidates for your attention. Give it some thought.

Also, I hope you appreciate the contributions that Arthur Jones has made to strength training. Without his insightful concepts and meaningful research, this book would be lacking in substance. Nautilus started a revolution in strength training during the 1970s. Bowflex is continuing with the message: *Your muscles matter most.* I'm grateful to be a part of both. And I'm pleased that you're strength training at home on Bowflex.

TOMORROW AND BEYOND

With your Bowflex machine and the routines in this book, you can *target, score, persist, win, and maintain* your body's leanness and strength.

May you thoroughly enjoy the adventure and the overall result: *Your New Bowflex Body.*

The Power Is Yours . . .

    Today,

        Tomorrow,

            and

                FOREVER!

Dr. Ellington Darden's BOWFLEX BODY PLAN

EXERCISE	Date						
	Body weight						
1.							
2.							
3.							
4.							
5.							
6.							
7.							
8.							
9.							
10.							
11.							
12.							

BIBLIOGRAPHY

Associated Press. "As Food Supply Gets Better, World Gets Fatter," *Orlando Sentinel*, February 4, 2001.

Barrett, Stephen, and Jarvis, William T. *The Health Robbers*. Buffalo, NY: Prometheus Books, 1993.

Baum, William et al. "A Nomogram for the Estimate of Percent Body Fat from Generalized Equations," *Research Quarterly for Exercise and Sport* 52: 380–84, 1981.

Bavley, Alan. "We Are the Fattest We Have Ever Been," *Orlando Sentinel*, October 27, 1998.

Beller, Anne Scott. *Fat and Thin: A Natural History of Obesity*. New York: Farrar, Straus and Giroux, 1977.

Benardot, Dan. *Nutrition for Serious Athletes*. Champaign, IL: Human Kinetics, 2000.

Bortz, Walter M. *We Live Too Short and Die Too Long*. New York: Bantam Books, 1991.

Brooks, Douglas. *Effective Strength Training*. Champaign, IL: Human Kinetics, 2001.

Campbell, W. et al. "Increased Energy Requirements and Changes in Body Composition with Resistance Training in Older Adults," *American Journal of Clinical Nutrition* 60: 167–75, 1994.

"Cereal: Best in the Bowl," *Consumer Report* 68: 29–33, September 2002.

Cooper, Kenneth A. *Aerobics*. New York: Bantam Books, 1968.

Darden, Ellington. *A Flat Stomach ASAP*. New York: Pocket Books, 1998.

———. *Body Defining*. Chicago: Contemporary Books, 1996.

———. *Two Weeks to a Tighter Tummy*. Dallas: Taylor Publishing, 1992.

———. *Hot Hips and Fabulous Thighs*. Dallas: Taylor Publishing, 1991.

———. *32 Days to a 32-Inch Waist*. Dallas: Taylor Publishing, 1990.

———. *BIG: The Ultimate Diet and Exercise Plan for Massive Muscles*. New York: Perigee Books, 1990.

———. *The Six-Week Fat-to-Muscle Makeover*. New York: G. P. Putnam's Sons, 1988.

———. *The Nautilus Diet*. Boston: Little, Brown and Company, 1987.

———. *The Nautilus Advanced Bodybuilding Book*. New York: Simon and Schuster, 1984.

———. *The Nautilus Bodybuilding Book*. Chicago: Contemporary Books, 1982.

———. *The Nautilus Nutrition Book*. Chicago: Contemporary Books, 1981.

———. *The Nautilus Book: An Illustrated Guide to Physical Fitness the Nautilus Way*. Chicago: Contemporary Books, 1980.

———. *Nutrition for Athletes: Myths and Truths*. Winter Park, FL: Anna Publishing, 1978.

———. *Nutrition and Athletic Performance*. Pasadena, CA: The Athletic Press, 1976.

———. "Frequently Asked Questions about Muscle, Fat, and Exercise," *Athletic Journal* 56: 20, 85–89, November 1975.

Davis, J. Mark et al. "Weight Control and Calorie Expenditure: Thermogenesis Effects of Pre-Prandial Exercise," *Addictive Behaviors* 14: 347–51, 1989.

Dupuis-Tate, Marie-France, and Fischesser, Bernard. *H2O: The Beauty and Mystery of Water*. New York: Harry N. Abrams, 2001.

Eller, Daryn. "20 Big Fat Diet Lies," *Family Circle* 106: 73–74, June 8, 1993.

Evans, William, and Rosenberg, Irwin, with Thompson, Jacqueline. *Biomarkers: The 10 Determinants of Aging You Can Control*. New York: Simon and Schuster, 1991.

Fiatarone, Maria A. et al. "High-Intensity Strength Training in Nonagenarians," *Journal of the American Medical Association* 263: 3029–34, 1990.

Food and Nutrition Board. *Recommended Dietary Allowances* (tenth edition). Washington, DC: National Academy Press, 1989.

Forbes, Gilbert B. *Human Body Composition: Growth, Aging, Nutrition, and Activity*. New York: Springer-Verlag, 1987.

———. "The Adult Decline in Lean Body Mass," *Human Biology* 48: 161–73, 1976.

Goldberg, Alfred L. et al. "Mechanisms of Work-Induced Hypertrophy of Skeletal Muscle," *Medicine and Science in Sports and Exercise* 7: 248–61, 1975.

Goldberg, Linn et al. "Changes in Lipid and Lipoprotein Levels after Weight Training," *Journal of the American Medical Association* 252: 504–06, 1984.

Gwinup, G. et al. "Thickness of Subcutaneous Fat and Underlying Muscles," *Annals of Internal Medicine* 74: 408–41, 1971.

Hales, Dianne. "What America Eats: What's Cooking at Your House?" *Parade,* November 11, 2001.

Hellmich, Nanci. "More Asians Believed Overweight," *USA Today*, March 17, 2003.

———. "Stress Can Put on Pounds," *USA Today*, January 2, 2002.

———. "Sleepless in America: More ZZZ's Needed," *USA Today*, March 25, 1998.

Howard, Pierce J. *The Owner's Manual for the Brain*. Austin, TX: Leornian Press, 1994.

Hutchins, Ken. *Super Slow: The Ultimate Exercise Protocol* (second edition). Casselberry, FL: Super Slow Systems, 1992.

International Health, Racquet and Sportsclub Association. *50 Million Members by 2010*. North Palm Beach, FL: Fitness Products Council, 1999.

Jones, Arthur. *The Lumbar Spine, the Cervical Spine, and the Knee*. Ocala, FL: MedX Corporation, 1992.

———. *Nautilus Training Principles: Bulletin No. 1*. DeLand, FL: Nautilus Sports/Medical Industries, 1970.

Katch, Frank I. et al. "Effects of Sit-up Exercise Training on Adipose Cell Size and Adiposity," *Research Quarterly for Exercise and Sport* 55: 242–47, 1984.

Keys, Ancel A. et al. "Basal Metabolism and Age of Adult Man," *Metabolism* 22: 579–87, 1973.

Kreider, Richard B. "Effects of Creatine Supplementation on Performance and Training Adaptations," *Molecular and Cellular Biochemistry* 244: 89–94, 2003.

Lamb, Lawrence E. *The Weighting Game*. Secaucus, NJ: Lyle Stuart, 1988.

Melby, C. et al. "Effect of Acute Resistance Exercise on Postexercise Energy Expenditure and Resting Metabolic Rate," *Journal of Applied Physiology* 75: 1847–53, 1993.

Messier, Stephen P., and Dill, Mary E. "Alterations in Strength and Maximal Oxygen Uptake Consequent to Nautilus Circuit Weight Training," *Research Quarterly for Exercise and Sport* 56: 345–51, 1985.

Mirkin, Gabe, with Foreman, Laura. *Getting Thin*. Boston: Little, Brown and Company, 1983.

Neergaard, Lauran. "Report: Obesity Can Harm Children," *Orlando Sentinel*, May 2, 2002.

———. "Satcher: Fat Kills Too Many Americans," *Orlando Sentinel*, December 14, 2001.

Nelson, Miriam E., and Wernick, Sarah. *Strong Women Stay Slim*. New York: Bantam, 1999.

Peterson, James A. "Total Conditioning: A Case Study," *Athletic Journal* 56: 40–55, September 1975.

Pollock, Michael L. et al. "Muscle," in *Rehabilitation of the Spine*, ed. Hochschuler, Richard D. et al. St. Louis: Mosby-Year Book, Inc., 1993.

Purvis, Tom. *Bowflex Ultimate: Owner's Manual & Fitness Guide*. Vancouver, WA: The Nautilus Group, 2002.

Raloff, Janet. "Vanishing Flesh: Muscle Loss in the Elderly Finally Gets Some Respect," *Science News*, August 10, 1996.

Roubenoff, Ronenn, and Castaneda, Carmen. "Editorial: Sarcopenia—Understanding the Dynamics of Aging Muscle," *Journal of the American Medical Association* 286: 1230–1231, 2001.

Rubin, Rita. "Lack of Sleep Feeds Men's Flab," *USA Today*, August 16, 2000.

Salamone, Debbie. "Florida's Water Crisis: The Human Thirst," *Orlando Sentinel*, April 7, 2002.

Shangold, Mona, and Mirkin, Gabe. *The Complete Sports Medicine Book for Women*. New York: Simon and Schuster, 1985.

Sizer, Frances S., and Whitney, Eleanor N. *Nutrition: Concepts and Controversies* (ninth edition), Belmont, CA: Wadsworth Publishing, 2003.

Smith, Kathy, with Miller, Robert. *Kathy Smith's Lift Weights to Lose Weight*. New York: Warner Books, 2001.

"The Truth about Dieting," *Consumer Reports* 67: 26–31, June 2002.

Vogel, Steven. *Prime Mover: A Natural History of Muscle*. New York: W. W. Norton & Company, 2001.

Wallenfels, Stephen. "CBI Interview: Brian R. Cook," *Club Business International* 23: 39–46, March 2002.

Westcott, Wayne. *Building Strength and Stamina* (second edition). Champaign, IL: Human Kinetics, 2003.

———. *Strength Fitness* (fourth edition). Dubuque, IA: William C. Brown Publishers, 1995.

Whitney, Eleanor N., and Rolfes, Sharon R. *Understanding Nutrition* (ninth edition). Belmont, CA: Wadsworth Publishing, 2001.

Winter, Greg. "Bigger Portions Are Supersizing Waistlines," *Orlando Sentinel*, July 7, 2002.

INDEX

cell characteristics, 123
   ability to increase, 124
   chemistry, 123
   consistency, 123
   gender differences, 124, 207
   number, 123, 129–30, 208
   as reproductive necessity, 124
   size, 123, 208, 210, 211
   storage location, 124, 207–8
   versatility, 124
cellulite, 208, 210
density of, 115
evolutionary reasons for, 121–23
ideal amount, 125
measuring, 124–25, 175–76
metabolic rate of, 116
percentage, 125, 125–26, 175–76
spot reduction, 211, 220–21, 271
Fat, dietary
   calories in, 140
   meal composition, 139
   physical stress from inadequate, 162
Fatigue, muscle, 116
Fat loss
   in Bowflex research study, 182
   effect of insulin on, 139–40
   nutrition, 136–41
   sleep effect on, 160–61
   strength training acceleration of, 9, 30
   stress effect on, 160, 162–63
   synergistic factors contributing to, 168–69
   water consumption and, 153–55
Fatty acids, 221
Fish, 254
Fly
   chest, 68, **68**, 229–30
   incline chest, **230**, 230–31
Food. *See also* Dieting; Eating plan; Meals; Menus; *specific foods*
   advertising by manufacturers, 120
   consumption per capita, 120
   dining out, 254
   fat in, 121
   holiday eating, 253–55
   portions, 120
   shopping list, 192–93

Food supplements
   creatine, 229, 232–35, 240–41, 272
   ergogenic aids, 147–48, 232
   meal replacements, 147
   minerals, 147, 178
   placebo effect of, 148
   protein, 143, 146–47
   regulation of, 143
   vitamins, 143, 147, 178
Frequency of training, 42, 47–49
Fruits, 192, 247, 253, 254

G

Genetics, of leanness, 129
Gluteals, exercises for, 58, **58**
Go Energy Shake, 147
Gorging, 121
Grains, 192
Guidelines
   for Bowflex use, 41–50
   for living leaner and stronger longer, 281
Gum, 247

H

Hamstrings, exercises for, 56, **56**, 58, **58**, 59, **59**
Hard-Body Challenge program, 195–96
   eating plan, 198–202
   maintenance guidelines, 205
   menus, 200–202
   results of participants, 199, **199**, 201, **201**, 204, **204**
   routines, 203–4
   strength training, 202–4
   success of, 196–98, 197, **197**
   superhydration, 204
Headaches, 267–68
Health clubs, 33, 36
Heat conservation, body size and, 128–29

M

Macaroni and cheese, 191
Machine components
    attachments, 21
    cables and pulleys, 21
    frame, 21
    hand grips/ankle cuffs, 21
    Power Rods, 19–20
    seat, bench, and platform, 21
Maintenance
    difficulty of, 258
    eating plan, 258, 260
    overlearning and, 262–64
    strength training, 261
    superhydration, 260
Meal replacements, 147
Meals
    composition, 139
    frequency, 140, 246, 260
    size, 139–40, 246, 260
Measuring, spoons and cups for, 178
Meat, 192. *See also specific meals;
        specific meats*
Menstruation, body fat and, 207
Menus
    Abdominal Focus program, 222–23
    Body-Leanness program, 189–92
    breakfast, 189, 200, 222
    dinner, 190–91, 200–202, 222–23
    Hard-Body Challenge program,
        200–202
    lunch, 189–90, 200, 222
    snacks, 190, 192, 200, 202, 222–23
Metabolism
    muscle mass effect on, 112, 116–17,
        276
    resting, 115–16
    strength training effect on, 9, 168
MET-Rx Drink Mix, 147
Mineral supplements, 147, 178
Momentary muscular failure, 43
Momentum, 44
Motivation, 183–84
Multiple-joint exercises, 100
Multiple sets, 43

Muscle, 112–14
    advantages of strong, 112
    belly shape, 216
    caloric demands of, 168, 247, 276
    fiber types, 116–17
    growth, 114
    hyperplasia, 114
    hypertrophy of, 114
    loss
        with age, 23
        atrophy, 114–17, 216, 280
        effect on metabolic rate, 116–17
        without strength training, 115
    order of working out, 42, 46–47
    over-developing, 216
    reduction with dieting, 31
    spot production, 211
    structure of, 114
    synergistic, 166
Muscular failure, momentary, 43
Muscular strength, 24
    evolutionary basis for, 163
    lower-body *vs* upper-body, 102
    negative and positive, 102
    effect of running on, 30
    starting level of, 98–99
Myoplex, 147

N

Nautilus equipment, 14
    Bowflex concept applied to, 36
    momentum on, 45
    revolution in strength training, 27–30
Negative-accentuated routines
    with Bowflex Leg Curl, 103–4
    with Bowflex Leg Extension, 103
    with Bowflex Leg Press Belt, 104
    thighs and calves, 106
    thighs and hips, 106–7
Negative-emphasized exercises
    seated biceps curl, 238–40, **239**
    seated triceps extension, 237–38, **238**
Negative phase, of a repetition, 101–4

ABOUT THE AUTHOR

Ellington Darden, Ph.D., has a goal: *to help people live leaner and stronger longer*. For the last 40 years he has worked with thousands of men and women who wanted to perform better physically, look more attractive, and improve overall health through a disciplined approach to nutrition and exercise.

He holds bachelor's and master's degrees in physical education from Baylor University and a doctorate in exercise science from Florida State University. Two years of postdoctoral study in food and nutrition set him on the trail that eventually led to *The Bowflex Body Plan*.

Dr. Darden was director of research for Nautilus Sports/Medical Industries for 20 years. There he helped develop and popularize the highly acclaimed Nautilus exercise equipment. Today, he resides with his wife, Jeanenne, and son, Tyler, in Orlando, where he continues with his training supervision and writing.

His outstanding research, which is applied in his books, is one of the reasons he was honored by the President's Council on Physical Fitness and Sports as one of the top ten health leaders in the United States. *The Bowflex Body Plan* is his 45th book. Contact Ellington Darden by going to www.Bowflex.com and then clicking on the "Ask Dr. Darden" banner.

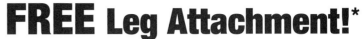

BOWFLEX®

FREE Leg Attachment!*

Get a FREE Leg Extension/Leg Curl Attachment – a $279 value – when you order a Bowflex Ultimate®

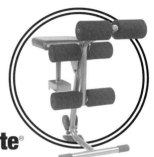

TAKE YOUR FITNESS TO A HIGHER LEVEL!

Maximize your results from *The Bowflex Body Plan* with the feature-packed Bowflex Ultimate:

MORE POWER:
- 310 lbs. of real Power Rod® resistance standard (upgradable to 410 lbs.)

MORE VERSATILITY:
- Over 90 exercises!

MORE CONFIDENCE:
- Industry-leading 10-YEAR Warranty!†

The Ultimate Full Body Workout Machine!™
Guaranteed Results in Just 6 Weeks!†

Bowflex Ultimate XLU

payments as low as
$55/mo.*

www.bowflexinfo.com

Call today:
(800) 269-5403